The Practical Patient

The Practical Patient

YOUR PERSONAL GUIDE THROUGH THE MEDICAL MAZE

Gail Zacok, MSN, RN, FNP-C

ISBN: 1544661444
ISBN 13: 9781544661445
Library of Congress Control Number: 2017903919
CreateSpace Independent Publishing Platform
North Charleston, South Carolina

Disclaimer

The medical and legal information in *The Practical Patient* is provided as an informational resource only, and is not to be used or relied on for any diagnostic or treatment purposes. This information does not create any patient-physician relationship, and should not be used as a substitute for professional diagnosis and treatment.

Never disregard professional medical advice or delay in seeking it because of something you have read in this book.

Be aware that, due to ongoing research and continuous changes in healthcare, information in *The Practical Patient* may be outdated.

The author expressly disclaims responsibility, and shall have no liability, for any damages, loss, injury, or liability whatsoever suffered as a result of your reliance on the information contained in this book.

Consult with your healthcare provider about any questions or concerns you may have on what you have read in *The Practical Patient*.

Table of Contents

INTRODUCTION

Navigating the Territory of Medicine

Wherever we go, whatever we do, and whomever we talk to, we encounter people who are sick. Many times they will talk about what is "wrong" with them, making it clear they do not really understand what it all means. Or, they will complain about their lack of time (or money) to get the proper healthcare, and feel they don't have any options. They will be frustrated with the medical machine - but unsure of what to do about it.

They will have many questions, but whom should they ask them of? Who can give them the answers they need, in a way they can understand?

We also can expect that at some point in our lives, each of us will become "the patient." For those of us who have had little experience with the healthcare system, maneuvering through the subsequent medical maze can be quite intimidating. Many times the unknowns - from scheduling an appointment to being a hospital patient - are overwhelming.

The territory of medicine is very similar to what it is like in a foreign country: the language is difficult to understand, the environment is unfamiliar, and the members of the community are busy doing their jobs while we, the visitors, try to figure out what is going on. It can be frightening if we have to enter such a country out of necessity, and especially if we are unprepared. When we end up having some sort of illness, not only must we cope with our condition and its often unpleasant, draining, and painful realities and symptoms, but we must also deal with some surroundings (be it in the hospital or the insurance company) that make little sense to us.

The Practical Patient is intended to direct and guide you through the health-care system so that you can be safe and secure while on your journey. If offers basic knowledge and insight into the often unpredictable world of medicine – knowledge and insight that is appropriate for all patients, regardless of age or illness. While *The Practical Patient* cannot address specific medical illnesses because of their specificity and complexity, it will help you to take your first steps toward improved health, a better patient-provider relationship, and peace of mind.

Dear Reader,

I know quite a few things about this "territory" - as I have lived in it for over thirty-six years. After twenty years of practicing as a registered nurse, I received my nurse practitioner's certification in family medicine. As of this writing, I continue to practice the art of nursing in a university clinic setting.

The Practical Patient offers health information to you in a down-to-earth and easily understandable manner. As you journey through the world of healthcare, *The Practical Patient* will give you a clearer understanding of what to expect. It will help you to know who your providers are and what their roles are, how to access these providers, and what to do when you see them. This book will offer both information and resources for illness prevention, screening for disease, and medication management. And finally, I will provide you with essential information on medical-legal topics and your rights as a patient.

I encourage you to bookmark pages, highlight passages, and fold over page corners. Scribble notes off to one side and share what you have learned with your family and friends. *The Practical Patient* will stimulate and preserve a positive relationship between you and your providers and give you the roadmap toward improved health.

Wishing you a happy and healthy life,

Gail, Nurse Practitioner

CHAPTER 1

Who the Providers Are
(While all physicians are doctors, not all doctors are physicians)

So what exactly does it mean to be a *patient*? You become a patient when a relationship has been established between you and a member of the medical community. Specifically, a relationship is formed when you demonstrate consent to being a patient by seeking medical services. In return, the healthcare provider consents to the relationship by examining, diagnosing, treating, or in some cases, agreeing to do so. This, though, does not apply in situations of extreme illness, when you are physically or mentally unable to make that decision. Healthcare will be provided to you, the patient, by a member of the medical community.

And there are many, many kinds of members whom you may run across.

Types of Physicians

There are two types of physicians - the Medical Doctor (MD) and the Doctor of Osteopathy (DO). Before reviewing these medical providers, let's first take a brief look at the history of healthcare and the evolution of physicians.

The art and science of healing dates back to prehistoric times, when plants, animal parts, and minerals were used to treat diseases. The first known physician in history is an Egyptian named Imhotep (2667 – 2648 BCE). Hippocrates, born on the Greek island of Kos in the fifth century BCE, is the most famous physician. He is credited with being the founder of modern medicine.

The practice of medicine in the United States (U.S.) dates back to colonial times – the early 1600s. At this time in history, England's practice of medicine was divided into three groups: the physicians (the "elite"; usually had a university degree), the surgeons (hospital-trained; often served the dual role of barber and surgeon), and the apothecaries (learned through an apprenticeship; prescribe, make, and sell medications). These distinctions did not survive in colonial America. In 1766, the New Jersey Medical Society was chartered, which began the process of regulating medical practice by setting educational standards, fee schedules, and a code of ethics.

Osteopathic medicine was founded in 1874 by Dr. Andrew Still, a physician and surgeon. Following the death of three of his children to spinal meningitis, he questioned the effectiveness of medical practices of his day, and concluded that the body contains all the essential features necessary to maintain health, if properly stimulated. Dr. Still believed the body's ability to heal itself could be greatly improved by the use of manual techniques, such as the manipulation of muscles and bones. Using this philosophy, Dr. Still opened the first school of osteopathic medicine in 1892 in Missouri. Osteopathic physicians use the diagnostic and therapeutic techniques of conventional medicine, as well as the use of *osteopathic manipulative treatment (OMT)* – the placement of hands on the body to diagnose, treat, and prevent illness or injury by using stretching, gentle pressure, and resistance techniques.

The MD and the DO have comparable educations:

a. Both have a Bachelor degree
b. Both must take the same test to get into their medical school programs – the Medical College Admissions Test (MCAT)
c. Both attend their respective schools of medicine for three to four years, depending on the program
d. Both must pass their respective examinations after completing medical school
   MD - *U.S. Medical Licensing Examination (USMLE)*
   ▪ Step 1 is usually taken at the end of the second year of medical school
   ▪ Step 2 is usually taken during the fourth year of medical school
   ▪ Step 3 is usually taken during the first or second year of Residency
   ▪ MD physicians must complete all three steps for medical licensure in the U.S.
   DO - *Comprehensive Osteopathic Medical Licensure Examination (COMLEX)*
   ▪ Level 1 is usually taken after completion of the second year of medical school
   ▪ Level 2 is usually taken during the third or fourth year of medical school
   ▪ Level 3 is usually taken after starting the Residency program
   ▪ The DO may also choose to take the USMLE, in place of the COMLEX. DO physicians must complete all three steps, of either test, for medical licensure in the U.S.

e. Once the MD and DO student have passed their exams, they are called *Physicians* or *Doctors*:

Tom Jones, MD (Medical Doctor/Doctor of Medicine) or Dr. Tom Jones
Mary Smith, DO (Doctor of Osteopathy) or Dr. Mary Smith

Following graduation from medical school, a setting that offers them exposure to all types of medicine and illnesses, the new physician chooses a medical specialty. They then attend a *"Residency"* program that focuses completely on that specialty.

Residency programs range from three to five years, depending on the specialty chosen. The first year of Residency is called the *"Internship"*, and during this time the new physician is commonly referred to as an *"Intern"*. A *"Resident"* refers to any physician in their Residency program. Once the physician has completed their Residency program and passes the certification test specific to that specialty, they are considered *"Board Certified"* in that field of medicine. According to the American Board of Medical Specialties, "Board Certification demonstrates a physician's exceptional expertise in a particular specialty and/or subspecialty of medical practice."

Examples of Residency programs follow. They include, but are not limited to:

- *Family Practice* / "General Practitioner" ("GP"): provides general healthcare to people of all ages
- *Pediatrics* / "Pediatrician": provides general healthcare to newborns up to eighteen to twenty-one years of age
- *Internal Medicine* / "Internist": provides general healthcare to adults from eighteen years of age and older

The three types of medical providers just referred to comprise the more general category of *"Primary Care Provider"* (PCP), a term used frequently in this book. This type of physician provides comprehensive healthcare to you as you age. They are responsible for coordinating your healthcare needs, as they:

- Identify and treat common medical conditions
- Provide preventive care (e.g., screenings and check-ups) and promote healthy lifestyle choices
- Assess the urgency of your medical problems and direct you to the best place for care
- Make referrals to medical specialists when necessary

A physician who specializes in a specific area of medicine is called a *"Specialist"*. Some well-known medical specialist Residency programs include: (*-ology* means "the study of"):

Anesthesiology / "Anesthesiologist":

- Gives general anesthesia before and/or during a surgical procedure (commonly referred to as, *"putting you to sleep"*)
- Offers *sedation* – intravenous (IV, or *into the vein*) medications to make the patient calm and/or unaware
- Injects *regional* anesthesia, or local anesthetic, near the nerves to "numb up" the part of the body being operated on

Dermatology / "Dermatologist":

- Diagnoses and treats diseases of the hair, skin, nails, and *mucous membranes* (the moist tissue that lines certain parts of the inside of your body, such as the nose, mouth, and lungs, and the urinary and digestive tracts)
- Performs skin surgery, such as removing skin cancer, to prevent or provide early control of disease
- Improves the skin's appearance by removing growths, discolorations, or damage caused by aging, sunlight, or disease
- Establishes a diagnosis through a *"biopsy"* – a procedure that removes a piece of tissue to be looked at under a microscope by a Pathologist

Neurology / "Neurologist":

- Diagnoses and treats disorders of the brain, spinal cord, and nerves

Obstetrics and Gynecology / "Gynecologist," "OB," or "OB/GYN":

- An Obstetrician is a physician who specializes in the management of pregnancy, labor, and the time period directly following childbirth

- A Gynecologist is a physician who specializes in the health of the female reproductive system
- Are trained in both Obstetrics and Gynecology
- Performs surgery when necessary

Ophthalmology / "Ophthalmologist":

- Diagnoses and treats diseases of the eye
- Performs eye surgery when necessary

Orthopedics / "Orthopedist":

- Diagnoses and treats conditions of the bones, joints, muscles, tendons, and ligaments
- Performs surgery when necessary
- Utilizes rehabilitation services, such as physical therapy

Pathology / "Pathologist":

- Studies body fluids and tissues, and can tell what is wrong with a patient, by studying the patient's cells under the microscope (resulting in, for example, a diagnosis of cancer)
- Performs autopsies to determine what caused an individual's death

Psychiatry / "Psychiatrist":

- Diagnoses, treats, and prevents mental health and emotional problems

Radiology / "Radiologist":

- Aids in the diagnosis of disease through x-ray, computerized tomography (CT), magnetic resonance imaging (MRI), positron emission tomography (PET), ultrasound, and nuclear medicine imaging techniques

- Treats abnormalities of the brain, spinal cord, or blood vessels
- Uses radiation to treat diseases, such as cancer

Surgery / **"Surgeon"**:

- Performs surgery (*"operations"*) to remove diseased tissue and organs (such as an appendix), replace diseased organs (such as a kidney transplant), and fix injuries (such as a broken bone)
- Provides care before, during, and after surgery

Urology / **"Urologist"**:

- Diagnoses and treats diseases involving the male and female urinary tract (kidneys and bladder), the male reproductive system, and the female pelvic floor (where the female reproductive parts rest)
- Performs surgery when necessary

Following Residency, the physician may then begin their medical practice or choose to focus on a more highly specific area of medicine by attending a *"Fellowship"* program, where they are known as *"Fellows"*. This takes an additional one to three years of study. After completing the Fellowship program, the Fellow must then pass their examination in order to receive certification. Examples of Fellowship programs include, but are not limited to:

- *Cardiology* / "Cardiologist": heart specialist
- *Critical Care Medicine* / "Intensivist": intensive care specialist; works in the Intensive Care Unit (ICU) where the patients are critically ill
- *Endocrinology* / "Endocrinologist": specialist of the endocrine system and hormones, treating such common conditions as diabetes and thyroid disease
- *Gastroenterology* / "Gastroenterologist": specialist in diseases of the digestive organs, ranging from the mouth and stomach to the intestines and anus; uses scopes to look into the stomach and colon
- *Geriatrics* / "Geriatrician": care of the elderly. (*Gerontology* is the study of aging and older adults)

- *Hematology* / "Hematologist": specialist in diseases of the blood
- *Hospice and Palliative Medicine*: "Palliative Specialist": specialist in end-of-life care. (*Palliate* means to relieve or lessen without curing)
- *Hospitalist*: specialist who gives comprehensive care to *only* the hospitalized patient
- *Infectious Disease* / "Infectious Disease Specialist": specialist in treating complicated and uncommon infections, such as HIV/AIDS
- *Neonatology* / "Neonatologist": specialist who cares for ill and/or premature newborns
- *Nephrology* / "Nephrologist": specialist in diseases of the kidney
- *Oncology* / "Oncologist": specialist in different types of cancer
- *Pediatrics* / "Pediatrician": specialist in treating newborns up to eighteen to twenty-one years of age. There are many sub-specialty areas within this field, including cardiology, critical care (intensive care), and surgery
- *Pulmonology* / "Pulmonologist": lung specialist
- *Psychiatry* / "Psychiatrist": specialist in mental health. There are many sub-specialties within this field, including Child and Adolescent, Geriatric (elderly), and Addiction
- *Rheumatology* / "Rheumatologist": specialist in autoimmune disorders and arthritis, and other diseases of the joints, muscles, and bones, such as lupus and rheumatoid arthritis
- *Surgery*: "Surgeon": specialist in a specific type of surgery, such as *thoracic* (chest organs - heart and lungs), pediatric (children), or plastic surgery
- *Traumatology* / "Traumatologist": trauma specialist

Nurse Practitioners and Physician Assistants

Although the educational process of the Nurse Practitioner (NP) and Physician Assistant (PA) is different (the specifics follow), the outcome is basically the same:

- Both must pass certifying exams
- Both have the option to do primary care or specialize
- Both are able to examine patients, prescribe medication, and order tests
- Both require continuing education to maintain certification
- Both are regulated by their individual state's governing board (although the laws from state to state vary)

Nurse Practitioner (NP)

The *Nurse Practitioner* (NP) movement began in 1965 by Loretta Ford, a nurse, and Dr. Henry Silver, who envisioned a nursing role that could assist families and children with access to affordable healthcare. Aware of the unmet health needs of poor communities, Ford felt confident that nurses could fulfill that need by providing healthcare in a professional capacity. Together, they created the first nurse practitioner training program at the University of Colorado (1965). As of June, 2017, there were over 234,000 licensed NPs in the U.S. and approximately 350 academic institutions with NP programs.

In order to enter a nurse practitioner program, the student must be a registered nurse (RN) and have a Bachelor of Science in Nursing (BSN) degree from an accredited educational institution. (*Author's Note:* A college or university is *accredited* when it has met a certain educational standard, set by a board of private educational associations. This ensures that the quality of education provided meets acceptable levels.)

The RN then applies to the NP program that specializes in their area of interest:

- *Adult-Gerontology Acute Care* (eighteen years to elderly; critical and/or complex chronic illnesses)
- *Adult-Gerontology Primary Care* (eighteen years to elderly; primary care)
- *Emergency Medicine*
- *Family Medicine* (newborn to elderly)
- *Neonatology* (premature infants)
- *Nurse Anesthetist* (anesthesia)
- *Nurse Midwife* (management of pregnancy and delivery)
- *Pediatrics Acute and/or Primary Care* (newborn to eighteen to twenty-one years of age)
- *Psychiatric-Mental Health*
- *Women's Health*

The NP program includes the advanced study of illnesses in the human body, how to recognize these illnesses, and how to medically manage these illnesses within the nurse's specialty. Upon completion, all graduates will have a Master of Science in Nursing (MSN) degree. The length of the NP program depends on the chosen specialty, full versus part-time student status, and whether or not the student already has a MSN degree. The nurse practitioner program generally takes eighteen to twenty-fours months to complete.

After completing the chosen specialty program, NPs must test and be certified by one of six certifying bodies:

1. American Academy of Nurse Practitioners
    Mary Smith, FNP-C (family nurse practitioner-certified)
        A-GNP-C (adult-gerontology nurse practitioner-certified)
        ENP-C (emergency nurse practitioner-certified)
2. American Nurses Credentialing Center
    Mary Smith, FNP-BC (family nurse practitioner-board certified)
        AGPCNP-BC (adult-gerontological primary care nurse practitioner-board certified)
        AGACNP-BC (adult-gerontological acute care nurse practitioner-board certified)
        PPCNP-BC (pediatric primary care nurse practitioner-board certified)
        PMHNP-BC (psychiatric-mental health nurse practitioner-board certified)
        ENP-BC (emergency nurse practitioner-board certified)
        (ANCC has retired testing for the following titles: Gerontological NP, Acute Care NP, School NP, and Adult NP. While new NPs can no longer receive this certification, NPs who already have these titles can continue to be recertified as long as the requirements are met.)
3. National Certification Corporation
    Mary Smith, WHNP-BC (women's health nurse practitioner-board certified)
        NNP-BC (neonatal nurse practitioner-board certified)
4. Pediatric Nursing Certification Board
    Mary Smith, CPNP-PC (certified pediatric nurse practitioner-primary care)
        CPNP-AC (certified pediatric nurse practitioner-acute care)
        CPNP-AC/PC (certified pediatric nurse practitioner-acute care/primary care)
5. National Board of Certification and Recertification for Nurse Anesthetists
    Mary Smith, CRNA (certified registered nurse anesthetist)
6. American Midwifery Certification Board
    Mary Smith, CNM (certified nurse-midwife)

A Nurse Practitioner is also known as a(n):

Advanced Care Practitioner (ACP)
Advanced Practice Nurse (APN)
Advanced Practice Registered Nurse (APRN)
Advanced Registered Nurse Practitioner (ARNP)
Certified Registered Nurse Practitioner (CRNP)

The highest degree obtainable for an NP is the Doctorate of Nurse Practitioner (DNP). It is not mandatory to have in order for the NP to practice medicine. A DNP is often recommended in healthcare administration and in the university setting. This degree gives the graduate the title of doctor:

Mary Smith, DNP (Doctorate of Nurse Practitioner) or Dr. Mary Smith

Each state has the authority to define the boundaries of practice for its resident nurse practitioners. Some states require that NPs have a contract with a physician, which is known as a Collaborative Practice Agreement (CPA). This document details the oversight of the NP by their collaborating physician. Other states allow NPs to practice medicine independently, without a CPA.

The NP's ability to know when to consult with or refer to a physician is developed in the educational arena and reinforced with hands-on experience. The NP is aware of their knowledge base and seeks assistance when their patient's health concern is outside of what they know, and/or when defined by the employer and/or state regulation.

Physician Assistant (PA)

The Physician Assistant (PA) profession began at Duke University by Dr. Eugene Stead. Like the nurse practitioner movement, their goal was to increase access to healthcare. The first students, former military medical corps veterans, graduated in 1967. In 2016, there were over 115,500 certified PAs and approximately 218 accredited PA programs.

The educational process of becoming a PA consists of twenty-four to thirty-six months of instruction at an accredited PA program. The first year is classroom studies. The second year is spent rotating through the different specialty areas. Most programs require the student to have a Bachelor degree for entrance and many programs award the student a Master degree upon graduation. (Author's Note: As of 2020, PA students must be awarded a Master degree as required by the PA Accreditation Review Commission.)

To obtain certification, the PA graduate takes an examination called the Physician Assistant National Certifying Exam (PANCE), which is administered by the National Commission on Certification of Physician Assistants.

Tom Jones, PA-C (physician assistant-certified)
Tom Jones, MPAS, PA-C (master of physician assistant studies, physician assistant-certified)

The PA-C may than chose to complete post-graduate clinical training that specialize in the areas listed below. Post-graduate studies are not required for PA licensure and practice:

- *Acute Care* (hospital-based)
- *Cardiology* (heart)
- *Cardiothoracic* (heart and lungs)
- *Critical Care/Trauma*
- *Emergency Medicine*
- *Family Medicine*
- *Geriatrics*
- *Hematology/Oncology* (diseases of the blood/cancer)
- *Hospitalist* (hospital-based)
- *Internal Medicine* (adult healthcare)
- *Neonatology*
- *OB/GYN*
- *Oncology*
- *Orthopedic surgery*
- *Otolaryngology (head and neck)*
- *Pediatrics*
- *Pediatric Neurology*
- *Primary Care*
- *Psychiatry*
- *Pulmonology*
- *Surgery*
- *Urgent Care*
- *Urology*

Each state has the authority to define the boundaries of practice for its resident physician assistants. However, all PAs practice medicine within the jurisdiction of a physician. Knowing when to consult with or refer to the physician is determined by the physician, employer, and/or state regulation.

Nurse Practitioners and Physician Assistants who specialize in *Family Medicine, Adult-Gerontology Care (primary care), Internal Medicine,* and *Pediatrics* are considered *Primary Care Providers (PCP)*. Like physicians, their job is to:

- Identify and treat common medical conditions
- Provide preventive care through screenings and check-ups, and promoting healthy lifestyle choices
- Assess the urgency of your medical problems and direct you to the best place for that care
- Make referrals to medical specialists when necessary

Additional Providers

Chiropractor

The student about to study chiropractic care typically has a Bachelor degree prior to entering the Doctor of Chiropractic (DC) program, which takes four to five years to complete. They obtain certification by passing the National Board of Chiropractors Examiners test.

Tom Jones, DC (Doctor of Chiropractic) or Dr. Tom Jones

Chiropractors care for patients with a wide range of injuries and disorders of the *musculoskeletal system* (muscles, ligaments, joints, and spinal cord) through manipulations or *chiropractic adjustments* – the use of hands or an instrument to manipulate the joints of the body in order to restore or enhance joint function. DCs also counsel patients on diet, nutrition, exercise, healthy habits, and occupational and lifestyle modifications.

Doctors of Chiropractic in New Mexico only are authorized to prescribe a limited number of medications. After receiving advanced education and certification through the American Chiropractic Physician Credentialing Center, the DC in New Mexico is referred to as a *Certified Advanced Practice Chiropractic Physician.*

Dentist

Prior to starting dental school, most prospective students have a Bachelor degree. Before being accepted into the dental program, they must take an entrance exam called the Dental Admission Test.

As in medical school, the first two years of dental school are spent in the classroom. During the second two years, the students have hands-on experience and rotate through the various specialties. Upon graduation, the student is awarded the degree of Doctor of Medicine in Dentistry/Doctor of Dental Medicine (DMD) or Doctor of Dental Surgery (DDS). It is up to the individual university to determine what degree is awarded. Both degrees use the same curriculum requirements set by the American Dental Association.

> *Mary Smith, DMD (Doctor of Medicine in Dentistry/Doctor of Dental Medicine) or Dr. Mary Smith*
> *Tom Jones, DDS (Doctor of Dental Surgery) or Dr. Tom Jones*

In order to be board-certified by the American Board of General Dentistry, the dental graduate must meet the three following requirements, per individual state guidelines:

- Educational: Graduate with a DDS or DMD degree from a program accredited by the Commission on Dental Accreditation
- Written: Pass the National Board Dental Examination
- Clinical: Demonstrate knowledge and dental skills by performing an oral examination

The dentist may then begin working in a dental practice, or they may choose to attend a Residency program for a more specialized area of study. These areas include:

- *Dental Public Health*: develops policies and programs that affect the community
- *Endodontics*: diagnoses and treats diseases and injuries that are specific to the dental nerves, pulp (the substance inside the tooth), and tissues that affect the health of the teeth (e.g., root canals)
- *Oral and Maxillofacial Pathology*: studies and researches the causes, processes, and effects of mouth and jaw diseases
- *Oral and Maxillofacial Radiology*: studies radiation physics, biology, safety, and hygiene related to the taking and interpretation of conventional and digital images, CT and MRI scans, and other imaging options
- *Oral and Maxillofacial Surgery*: provides diagnostic services and treatments for diseases, injuries, and defects of the neck, head, jaw, and associated structures (for example, through dental implants, wisdom teeth removal, or surgery for head and neck cancers)

- *Orthodontics and Dentofacial Orthopedics*: treats problems related to irregular dental development, missing teeth, and other abnormalities (for example, braces, headgear, and retainers)
- *Pediatric Dentistry*: specializes in children's dentistry
- *Periodontics*: diagnoses and treats diseases of the gums, mucous membranes, tissues that surround and support the teeth, and bone supporting the teeth, such as through dental implants and surgical procedures for severe gum disease
- *Prosthodontics*: replaces missing natural teeth with fixed or removable appliances, such as dentures, bridges, and implants

Licensed Counseling Services

A *Licensed Counselor* is trained to prevent, diagnose, and manage mental health and emotional problems. The educational requirements, titles, licensing guidelines, and practice restrictions are regulated by each individual state. A licensed counselor can work in all areas of healthcare including hospitals, private practice, and school settings. There are also a wide variety of sub-specialties within this field, including:

- *Child Mental Health*
- *Adult Mental Health*
- *Learning Disabilities*
- *Emotional Disturbances*
- *Substance Abuse*
- *Geriatrics (elderly)*

A *Licensed Clinical Psychologist (LCP)* holds a Doctorate degree in psychology or philosophy. They are able to practice independently, meaning they are able to provide counseling services without oversight. As of this writing, with additional training, LCPs can prescribe medication in Louisiana, New Mexico, Illinois, Idaho, Iowa, in the military, and in the Indian Health Service.

Tom Jones, PsyD (Doctor of Psychology) or Dr. Tom Jones
Mary Smith, PhD (Doctor of Philosophy) or Dr. Mary Smith

Just as the educational and licensing requirements vary from state to state, so do the titles counselors can have. Listed below are examples of some of the possible counseling titles. Licensing bodies include the National Clinical Mental Health Counseling Examination and the National Counselor Examination for Licensure and Certification:

- *Licensed Clinical Professional Counselor (LCPC)*
- *Licensed Professional Counselor (LPC)*
- *Licensed Mental Health Counselor (LMHC)*
- *Licensed Professional Clinical Counselor (LPCC)*
- *Licensed Mental Health Counselor (LMHC)*
- *Licensed Professional Counselor (LPC)*

Examples of *Marriage and Family* counselor titles include:

- *Marriage and Family Therapist (MFT)*
- *Licensed Marriage and Family Therapist (LMFT)*
- *Medical Family Therapist Associate (MFTA)*
- *Licensed Associate Marriage and Family Therapist (LAFMT)*

Examples of *Specialized* Certification include:

- School
- Rehabilitation
- Addiction
- Pastoral
- Expressive Arts Therapies; Music Therapy; Dance/Movement Therapy
- Christian counseling

Licensed Clinical Social Worker

Before becoming *a Licensed Clinical Social Worker (LCSW)*, the student first must graduate with a Master of Social Work (MSW). Upon graduating with a MSW, the student then is eligible to obtain the title of *Licensed Master Social Worker (LMSW)* by passing the first of two tests via the Association of Social Work Boards (ASWB).

At this level, the LMSW and MSW (their requirements varying from state to state) help people solve and cope with problems in their everyday lives. They may work with children, people with disabilities, and people with serious illnesses and addictions. Their job responsibilities are to:

- Identify people who need help
- Assess clients' needs, situations, strengths, and support networks to determine their goals
- Develop plans to improve their clients' well-being
- Help clients adjust to changes and challenges in their lives, such as illness, divorce, or unemployment
- Research and refer clients to community resources, such as food stamps, child care, and healthcare
- Help clients work with government agencies (such as Medicare and Medicaid) to apply for and receive benefits
- Respond to crisis situations, such as child abuse
- Advocate for, and help clients get, resources that would improve their well-being
- Follow-up with clients to ensure that their situations have improved
- Evaluate the services being provided to ensure that they are effective

In order to earn the distinction of *Licensed Clinical Social Worker (LCSW)* the LMSW must put in an additional 2,000 - 4,000 hours in supervised clinical counseling over two years (the number of hours vary from state to state). They then must take a second test via the ASWB. In addition to having the job duties of a LMSW, the Licensed Clinical Social Worker (LCSW) is certified to work independently in counseling roles with families, individuals and children, work in school intervention situations, provide therapeutic counseling in hospital settings, and open their own practice as a counselor or therapist.

Optometrist

The optometrist typically has a Bachelor degree prior to entering the Doctor of Optometry program. Applicants must take the Optometry Admission Test (OAT) prior to entering the program, which takes four years to complete. Certification is given by the National Board of Examiners in Optometry.

Mary Smith, OD (Doctor of Optometry) or Dr. Mary Smith

Upon passing the certification test, the optometrist has the option to enter into an optometry practice or complete a residency program for specialized training, such as in diseases of the eye or brain injury vision rehabilitation.

The optometrist's responsibilities include:

- Examining the eyes and other parts of the visual system
- Diagnosing and treating visual problems
- Managing diseases, injuries, and other disorders of the eyes
- Prescribing eyeglasses, contact lenses, and medications

For review, an *ophthalmologist* is a medical doctor who specializes in diseases of the eye. This includes the diagnosis and treatment of eye illness and injury, and performing eye surgery. An *optometrist* can examine the eye, treat diseases of the eye, and prescribe eyeglasses, contact lenses, and medication. *Opticians* are technicians trained to design and fit eyeglass lenses and frames, contact lenses, and other devices to correct eye sight.

Pharmacist

Prior to attending a Doctor of Pharmacy program, a student must have at least two years of undergraduate study, although some programs require a Bachelor degree. Most programs also require applicants to take the Pharmacy College Admissions Test (PCAT).

The Doctor of Pharmacy program typically takes four years to complete. The pharmacist graduate then must pass two exams to be licensed and receive the title of *Doctor of Pharmacy (PharmD)*:

1. The North American Pharmacist Licensure Exam (NAPLEX), which tests pharmacy skills and knowledge
2. The Multistate Pharmacy Jurisprudence Exam (MPJE) or a state-specific test on pharmacy law

Tom Jones, PharmD (Doctor of Pharmacy) or Dr. Tom Jones

The graduate Pharmacist has the option to begin work as a Pharmacist or attend a two-year Residency program. The first year enhances the skills of a general pharmacist in healthcare systems, managed care, and community settings. Year two provides advanced training in a focused area of patient care, such as Emergency Medicine, Infectious Disease, or Pediatrics.

A pharmacist is responsible for:

- Regulating the quality and quantity of medicines
- Dispensing medicines
- Educating and advising patients regarding their medicine
- A pharmacist cannot prescribe medications, but is licensed to give vaccinations pending individual state law and company policy

Podiatrist

A *Doctor of Podiatric Medicine (DPM)* specializes in the prevention, diagnosis, and treatment of conditions of the foot, ankle, and related structures of the lower leg resulting from injury or disease. A DPM makes independent judgments, prescribes medications, and performs surgery.

To enter a school of podiatric medicine, the student must first complete a minimum of three years or ninety semester hours of college credit. Standardized testing requirements before admission vary among schools. They include the:

- MCAT (Medical College Admissions Test)
- GRE (Graduate Record Examination)
- DAT (Dental Admissions Test)

The Doctor of Podiatric Medicine (DPM) study is four years in length. The first two years are devoted to classroom studies. The second two years concentrate on clinical experience. Upon graduation, the student must then pass the American Podiatric Medical Licensing Exam.

Podiatrists must then complete a Residency program. The podiatric medicine and surgery residency program consists of three years of training in inpatient (hospital) and outpatient (community) medical and surgical management. The American Board of Foot and Ankle Surgery and the American Board of Podiatric Medicine are the certifying boards for this field.

Mary Smith, DPM (Doctor of Podiatric Medicine) or Dr. Mary Smith

CHAPTER 2

Finding A Provider
(But what if I don't want to be a patient?)

The benefits of establishing with a Primary Care Provider (PCP) before getting sick or injured are many:

- The PCP and you will have already met, and so you're familiar with each other. This helps to reduce any stress levels you may have when you need to be seen for an illness or injury appointment
- The PCP already knows your medical history. If you are not feeling well, or if an illness has caused your mind to be a bit fuzzy about your health history, it will not hamper your provider's exam, diagnosis, and treatment of your case
- It is quite reassuring to know that you have someone available to you should you become ill or injured
- There is an additional ease to scheduling appointments with a PCP when a relationship is already in place. It takes less time, and is less stressful to conduct
- Any questions about paperwork, insurance, money, and clinic location and hours have already been worked out

So taking the time to find a PCP before you need one will not only help you to keep focusing on your health, but it will save you time and energy when you are sick and in need of prompt medical attention.

Yet all too often, people do not look for medical help until they are in actual need of it. The reasons for this are many. (Do any of these reasons sound familiar?)

- "I live a healthy lifestyle, so I don't need to see a provider. I watch what I eat, and I exercise, too."
- "Who has the time? I'm too busy handling my job and the kids."
- "Finances are tight right now. I don't have the money to go see someone."
- "Providers don't know what they're doing! Every day we're finding out about some medicine they said would help us can actually kill us!"
- "I know I should go see someone, but there are so many provider and clinic choices. I don't know where to go, or who I should see for my condition."
- "I see someone in my insurance network, but I don't like them. They treat me like a number, and they think they know everything. They never listen to what I have to say."
- "I'd go see someone, but I can't find a ride."
- "What are they going to tell me that I don't already know?"
- "Why go? They'll just find out more things wrong with me."

When people desire to establish a relationship with a PCP and practice preventive healthcare, they discover they share a common goal with their PCP - to improve their health and prolong their life by:

- Finding diseases, many times before there are symptoms, and treating them sooner
- Receiving vaccines that prevent illness, disability, and death
- Learning and practicing healthy lifestyle habits
- Having regular check-ups

Preventive (or Preventative) care is the care you receive to prevent illness and disease. And for those with insurance, it makes financial sense too. In the majority of healthcare insurance plans, preventive health services are covered 100 percent and require no out-of-pocket costs (*see Chapter 7 for Preventive Health services*)

Whether or not you choose to keep a careful eye on your health, there comes a point in time when you (along with everyone else on the planet) need medical care, whether you want to have it - or not. This generally happens in one of three ways: through a health clinic, through the Urgent Care, or through the Emergency Room (also called the *ER, Emergency Department, ED*). With each scenario, once a life-threatening emergency has been ruled out, the staff will ask you (or those accompanying you) right away about whether or not you have health insurance, and if so, what type is it. To help you out with understanding your healthcare situation, I will run through the basics in terms of how insurance plans are structured and their common terminology, so you can gain a good general understanding of it.

Because the politics of health insurance are in a constant state of change, it does not make sense for me to focus on the countless details of the many available plans. If you have specific questions about your plan, contact your insurance agent – although do it now, rather than waiting until you are in more urgent need.

After we discuss health insurance plan basics, I'll go about discussing how you can best establish a relationship with a provider.

Health Insurance Plan Basics

Here are some of the more common terms used in the health insurance industry that will apply to the health coverage you may have:

- *Deductible*: A fixed dollar amount that an insured person pays before the insurance company starts to make payments for "covered" medical services. The amount you pay out-of-pocket, and how much of that money your insurance company applies toward your deductible, may vary if services are received from an approved (in-network; *see below*) provider versus an out-of-network provider. Some in-network services may be covered by your insurance company before you have met your deductible. The deductible benefit period is typically for one year
- *Co-insurance*: the percentage of money you pay for each healthcare service, office visit, and prescription after you have paid your deductible. Know that you may be responsible for any charges *in excess* of what the insurance company determines to be "*usual, customary, and reasonable*" (UCR), which is the cost amount an insurance carrier is willing to pay for a specific service. (The UCR cost amount is based on what providers in your area usually charge for the same or similar medical service)
- *Co-pay* (co-payment): the fixed amount you pay for each healthcare service provided, such as an office visit or a prescription. There may be different co-pay amounts for different services, such as for a visit to an Urgent Care or

Emergency Room. Some plans may require you to meet your deductible before the co-pay option applies
- *Premium*: the fee you agree to pay for coverage of medical benefits in a defined period of time. For example, every two weeks your employer deducts the same insurance premium from your paycheck
- *Maximum out-of-pocket*: the most you will have to pay for covered medical expenses in a plan year. The maximum is reached through deductible, coinsurance, co-payment, and out-of-pocket contributions. Once you have paid the maximum out-of-pocket, your insurance plan begins to pay 100 percent of *covered* medical expenses for the remainder of the plan year
- *(In-)Network*: a group of physicians, hospitals, and other healthcare providers that agree to provide medical services at pre-negotiated rates with your insurance company
- *Explanation of Benefits (EOB)*: statement from your insurance company that summarizes the billed charges from all the providers and medical facilities, payments made by your insurance company, prescription payments, and the estimate of what is owed by you. (Keep in mind this is just a summary and not the actual bill)

As a general rule: The higher your deductible = the lower your premium = the more you will initially pay out-of-pocket for healthcare services (to meet your deductible). The lower your deductible = the higher your premium = the less you will pay out of pocket to meet your deductible (but you will be paying more in premiums).

Managed Care Organizations (MCO)

Managed Care Organizations (MCOs) are organizations that combine the functions of health insurance, delivery of healthcare, and administration into one package. It is a healthcare delivery system consisting of hospitals, physicians, and other services which provide a wide range of coordinated health services. MCO is an umbrella term for health plans that provide healthcare in return for a predetermined monthly fee and coordinate care through a defined network of physicians and hospitals.

MCOs contract directly with *healthcare providers and health systems* - the plan's *network* - to provide care for a plan's members at a reduced cost. By providing a wide variety of quality healthcare services to enrolled workers, they are able to keep medical costs down. How much of your healthcare your plan will pay for depends on your insurance company and the rules of the network. Plans that limit your choices usually cost less. More flexible plans may cost more.

There are four major types of managed care plans:

- *Health Maintenance Organizations (HMO)* usually only pay for care *within the network*. You must choose a primary care provider (PCP) in the network who will coordinate most of your care. For example, if you wish or need to see a specialist, you must obtain a referral from your PCP first. Seeing a provider outside of the network is usually not covered by this type of insurance. A referral is usually not needed to see an in-network Obstetrician/Gynecologist
- *Preferred Provider Organizations (PPO)* allow for more flexibility in your choice of providers, as compared to a HMO. In this type of plan, you can visit any in-network healthcare provider without obtaining a referral from your PCP. Staying inside the network costs you, as a member, less. You may seek healthcare outside of the network without a referral, but this costs more
- *Point of Service (POS)* plans are a combination of the HMO and PPO. With this plan, you must choose a PCP. If the PCP refers you to a specialist in the network, your costs will be lower. If you choose to see a provider outside of the network, your costs will be higher
- *Exclusive Provider Organizations (EPO)* are a more restrictive type of plan in which you must use providers from a specific network. You won't need to choose a primary care provider, and you don't need referrals to see a specialist. There is no coverage for care received outside of the network, except in cases of emergency

Medicare and Medicaid are examples of Managed Care Organizations (MCOs). They provide health benefits and other services through contracted arrangements between state agencies and MCOs that accept a fixed amount of payment for services.

In general, Medicare is available to most people aged sixty-two years and older. It is a federally-administered program available to those who meet *all* the following criteria:

1. At least sixty-two years of age,
2. U.S. citizen or permanent legal resident with five years of continuous residence, and
3. They, or their spouse, have worked at a job where they paid Medicare taxes for at least ten years.

Medicare helps to cover the cost of services for healthcare in four ways:

1. *Part A: Hospital insurance*
    ▪ Inpatient care in hospitals
    ▪ *Skilled* nursing facility, such as a nursing home, for certain *medically-nec-essary* conditions for a limited time. (Healthcare services or supplies are "*medically necessary*" if they are needed to diagnose or treat an illness or injury, condition, disease, or its symptoms. These services must meet accepted medical standards and are determined by each insurance company. Medicare does not cover nursing home or home health *custodial* care, such as assistance with bathing or dressing)
    ▪ Hospice care
    ▪ Home healthcare that is medically-necessary
2. *Part B: Medical insurance*
    ▪ Healthcare providers
    ▪ Outpatient care
    ▪ Durable medical equipment, such as wheelchairs and nebulizers
    ▪ Some preventive services
3. *Part C: Medicare Advantage*
    This allows private Medicare-approved health insurance companies to provide *additional* Medicare benefits and coverage. These plans include all the benefits and services covered under Parts A and B.
4. *Part D: Medicare prescription drug coverage (attached to Part C coverage)*

For further questions, visit the Medicare website: www.medicare.gov. For questions about cost, visit www.medicare.gov/your-medicare-costs/costs-at-a-glance/costs-at-glance.html.

Medigap insurance, also known as *Medicare supplement insurance,* is a separate policy that can be bought from private health insurance companies to help cover some of the gaps in Medicare coverage, such as co-payments, co-insurance, and deductibles.

Medicaid, a MCO available to the very young and old, offers benefits limited to U.S. citizens and lawfully-present immigrants who have lived in the U.S. for at least five years (although individual states can eliminate the waiting period for pregnant women and children).

Individual states can set the eligibility criteria within federal minimum standards. According to Medicaid.gov:

"States establish and administer their own Medicaid programs and determine the type, amount, duration, and scope of services within broad federal guidelines. States are required to cover certain "mandatory benefits," and can choose to provide other "optional benefits" through the Medicaid program."

Examples of mandatory benefits include inpatient hospital services, outpatient clinic services, childhood physicals and screenings, home health services, lab and x-ray services, and family planning services. Optional benefits include physical and occupational therapy, optometry and dental services, and Hospice care.

In order for states to receive federal funding that covers part of the cost of running the Medicaid program, they must include coverage to the following core group of individuals:

- Children through age eighteen in families with an income below 138 percent of the federal poverty level
- Pregnant women with an income below 138 percent of the federal poverty level
- Certain low-income parents
- Most seniors and persons with disabilities who receive financial assistance through the Supplemental Security Income (SSI) program

Because individual states have the flexibility to cover others *above* the mandatory limits (and thereby receive additional federal funds), eligibility varies significantly from state to state.

Accountable Care Organizations (ACO)

The Medicare *Shared Savings Program* (SSP) is a key component of the Medicare delivery system reform initiatives included in the Affordable Care Act. Congress created the SSP to facilitate coordination and cooperation among providers to improve the quality of care for Medicare Private Fee-For-Service (PFFS) beneficiaries and reduce unnecessary costs. Eligible providers, hospitals, and suppliers participate in the Shared Savings Program by creating or participating in an Accountable Care Organization. (PFFS: a type of Medicare Advantage Plan [Part C] offered by a private insurance company.)

Accountable Care Organizations (ACO) are groups of doctors, hospitals, and other healthcare providers who *voluntarily* come together to give coordinated, high-quality care to their patients. The Shared Savings Program will reward ACOs that lower their growth in healthcare costs while meeting performance standards on quality of care and putting patients first. The goals of ACOs are to:

- make sure that patients get the right care at the right time
- avoid repeating services
- prevent medical errors
- encourage quality improvement and care coordination resulting in better care, smarter spending, and healthier people
- set clear, measurable goals and a timeline toward paying providers based on the quality of the care given, rather than on the number of patients to whom care is given to
- set predictable financial targets, which allows both providers and patients greater opportunities to coordinate care
- attain the highest quality standards of care
- improve communication between patients, their providers, and other healthcare services

ACOs can be found in the commercial health insurance industry, Medicare, and Medicaid. By end of March, 2017, there were 923 active ACOs across the U.S. covering 32 million lives. Medicare ACOs in your area can be found at the following website:
data.cms.gov/ACO/2016-Medicare-Shared-Savings-Program-Accountable-C/i683-k66m.
Medicaid ACOs can be found at the following website:
www.chcs.org/resource/medicaid-aco-state-update/.

Now let's look at how to establish a relationship with a provider in different settings, and what it is going to cost you.

Health Clinics and Establishing With a Provider

Searching for a provider can be exhausting and stressful. Quickly finding someone who is trustworthy and knowledgeable may seem challenging, but there are things you can do to make it easier. And when looking for a provider, the first thing many households have to consider is cost. This involves looking at your type of insurance or your lack of insurance, and any potential out-of-pocket costs.

For Those With Insurance

Begin by carefully reviewing your plan to see what local healthcare systems are covered (in-network) in your area before you need to use them. Here I am referring to healthcare systems, medical clinics, Urgent Care facilities, and hospital Emergency Rooms. The very next step is to then determine what you must pay out of pocket before the insurance company starts to pay. This could include both a *deductible* and a *co-pay*. Remember that the co-pay can vary in cost if your visit is to a clinic, an Urgent Care facility, or an Emergency Room. Staying within your network will decrease, but not necessarily eliminate, your out-of-pocket costs.

The quickest and easiest way to see what providers and health clinics are covered is to go to your insurance company's website and search for a provider or health system near you. The address of this website can usually be found on the back of your insurance card. Or, you can do an Internet search for the name of the insurance company, which usually will bring up the respective website.

Once you reach the site, you may need to register in order to do a search within the website. After entering the requested information, the search will come back to you with names, specialties, addresses, and phone numbers of those providers and healthcare systems that are in-network. Some websites will post a picture of the provider and a brief paragraph about their medical education along with the local hospitals they are affiliated with. While there may be multiple listings of providers within your network, this does not mean all of them are accepting new patients. When at the insurance website, look to see if there is a listing of *only* the providers who are accepting new patients should you be looking for a new provider.

Your insurance card may include a *"Member Services"* telephone number, which can be helpful to you in finding a local covered provider or healthcare system, and for answering any other questions you may have. If you call this number, have your insurance identification and/or group number handy. This information can be found on the front of your insurance card. The insurance representative may also ask for your address and date of birth to help confirm your identity.

Once you have determined what healthcare systems are in-network, go to that healthcare systems' website. Click the tab for "local providers", or something similar. Usually, but not always, if the healthcare system is in-network, so are the providers in that healthcare system.

If you know what clinic you want to go to, call it and ask if they accept your certain type of insurance. Doing an Internet search may or may not be helpful. While this search can quickly locate providers, the information can be outdated and unreliable.

Be aware that it is common for new providers and providers who are accepting new patients to advertise in the local newspaper.

It is important to note that some health insurance policies can only be used in certain states. If you traveling to or attending school in a state other than your residence, check to see if your insurance benefits can be used in that state. And if so, look to see what Urgent care facilities and hospital healthcare systems are considered in-network, in case of an emergency.

When it comes to Medicare, there is a specific governmental website to search for providers and/or hospitals in your area: *www.medicare.gov/physiciancompare/search.html.*

For Those Without Insurance

When you don't have insurance, you are not so much restricted by which provider you can see, but by how much money you can afford to spend. Know that there are medical clinic options for you.

There are two primary types of clinics: those owned by a healthcare system (providers are employees of the system) and those that are independently owned. Either may be a solo practice (only one provider) or a group practice. Some will have Electronic Health Record (EHR) technology, some will not (this will be reviewed in Chapter 3). Both will most likely have contracts with certain health insurance companies. Both will have a *self-pay* (cash-pay) policy.

If you have no insurance but want to see a specific clinic provider, you can call that clinic and ask what their self-pay policy is. Generally, for the first office visit, many clinics will require a cash-up-front amount of money. Some may require a contract to be signed regarding payment being made within a specified amount of time. Once you, the self-pay patient, understand what is expected, you will be better able to decide if you want and (can afford) to go to that clinic. You may also ask the clinic if it has any information or resources available that will assist you in obtaining insurance or financial assistance.

Another clinic option for the self-pay patient is a *federally-funded* (government funded) healthcare clinic or a *healthcare-system-affiliated* (healthcare system-supported) healthcare clinic for the uninsured. These types of clinics are specifically designed for patients with no or inadequate insurance coverage. Commonly, such clinics base their payment fees on patient income using a *"sliding-scale system"* - which means the cost of the office visit is based from how much you earn. You may need to provide proof of current residency, a photo ID and/or birth certificate, last year's federal tax return, and/or proof of income when the appointment is made. There may also be a standard fee regardless of income.

These clinics may have information or resources available that will assist you in obtaining insurance. The U.S. government has a website to help patients in finding a government-based clinic close and convenient to them: *findahealthcenter.hrsa.gov.*

For additional options, contact your local Health Department to see what health services are available to you as a resident. Funding sources for these clinics come from federal funds, state and local funds, and county and city revenues. Their services may be at no cost to you, the fee may be based on a sliding-scale, there may be a charge per service depending on what your needs are, or your insurance may be billed. Because the Health Department funding varies from state to state, there may be certain services offered in one state but not in another. Some local Health Department clinic options may include:

- *Family Planning:* sexually transmitted disease screening and treatment, female exams, birth control
- *Women, Infant, and Children (WIC):* supplemental foods, healthcare referrals, and nutrition education for low-income pregnant women, breastfeeding and non-breastfeeding women after giving birth, and for infants and children up to age five who are found to be at nutritional risk
- *Immunizations:* child and adult vaccines; travel vaccines
- *Assistance with finding health insurance and healthcare*

Regardless of whether you do or do not have insurance, you can't ask too many questions when searching for a provider. To end this section, I encourage you to consider the following additional questions in your quest:

- Are they accepting new patients?
- How soon can I be seen?
- Are the office hours convenient for you?
- Are evening or weekend appointments available?
- Is the office at a convenient location?
- Is it easy to get there?
- Is it close to any form of public transportation?
- Is parking free and available if you drive there?
- Is it handicap-accessible?

- What forms of payment are accepted? (Some clinics only accept cash and checks regardless of your insurance status)
- If you need a translator, is one available?

Urgent Care and Emergency Rooms

The unexpected has now happened... and you need to see a provider *right away.*

If you have a PCP, you should call their office first. If the problem can be managed there, they will make arrangements for you to be seen. If the problem can't be managed there, they will advise you on what to do next. If you call the PCP after-hours, listen for instructions after the initial message. Some offices will have a provider on-call for you to talk to, while others may refer you to a local and/or specific Urgent Care or Emergency Room.

If you have insurance, some companies offer a twenty-four hour Nurse Hotline telephone number for health questions. The insurance plan's website will contain this information. The back of your insurance card may have the Nurse Hotline number listed, or you can call the insurance company's Customer Service for the information.

If your problem can't be managed at home or at your provider's office, it is time to think about going to the Urgent Care or to the Emergency Room. Regardless of whether you have a primary care provider (PCP) and insurance or not, going to the Urgent Care or the Emergency Room can be a difficult decision. Trying to decide if your illness can wait or if you need to go right away can challenge most people.

(*Author's Note:* Know that if you decide to go the Emergency Room and your insurance company does not consider your illness or injury to be an emergency, some insurance companies can deny payment to the Emergency Room, who will then bill you.)

If you think it can wait, make an appointment as soon as possible with your PCP. If not, the next decision you should make is if to go to the Urgent Care or the Emergency Room. Keep in mind that some Urgent Care centers and Emergency Rooms allow you to see how long the wait time is and/or schedule an appointment on their websites. To also assist you in making this essential decision, I am going to list the major differences between the Urgent Care and the Emergency Room:

1. *Urgent Care characteristics*:
    - Usually open after normal business hours, including evenings and weekends
    - Designed to treat non-life threatening injuries, such as cuts and minor injuries, and illnesses, such as earaches, the flu, and rashes
    - May offer on-site diagnostic tests, such labs, x-ray, and CT
    - Less expensive for both co-payment and out-of-pocket costs
    - Shorter waiting times (generally)
    - Often provide general healthcare, including vaccines and physicals for school or sports
2. *Emergency Room characteristics*:
    - Open and staffed twenty-four hours a day, seven days a week
    - Designed to treat patients suffering from life-threatening injuries and serious illnesses
    - Have the widest range of services for emergency after-hours health-care, including diagnostic testing (lab, x-ray, CT) and access to specialists
    - Because the Emergency Room is usually located within a hospital, there is a smooth transfer if the patient needs to be hospitalized
    - Longer wait times (generally)
    - Generally more expensive for both co-payment and out-of-pocket costs

If you have been seen in the Urgent Care or Emergency Room and require a follow-up office visit, the facility will most likely give you a provider name and phone number at your discharge, if you do not already have one. This may be a primary care provider or specialist, depending on the type of illness or injury for which you were seen. Know that in most cases, you will be responsible for making the appointment. It is important for you to schedule the recommended follow-up appointment for the following reasons:

- To decide whether to continue the treatment you received,
- To make sure you received the correct diagnosis and treatment,
- To make changes if you haven't gotten better or have gotten worse, or
- To decide what to do if you didn't follow the discharge instructions, and continue to not feel well.

Here are more points to consider when choosing a provider after you've been seen in the Urgent Care or Emergency Room:

- If you choose to use a different provider other than the name given to you at the Urgent Care or Emergency Room, you are free do so. But if you do so, look to see if they are covered by your health insurance plan (with insurance) or call to see what their self-pay policy is (without insurance)
- If you are being referred to the specialist who treated you in the Emergency Room, consider following up with that specialist as you and they have already met, and they are familiar with your health problem. Also, it may be easier to schedule an appointment as you have already seen this provider in the ER and were specifically referred to them
- If you have insurance and choose to go out of network, you will be responsible for paying the amount of money not covered by insurance
- It is important to remember that the Urgent Care and the Emergency Room are designed to take care of your immediate problem, and then, if it is needed, they will refer you to someone who will continue to care for you until your health problem is better. Your primary care provider may be able to continue treating you, or you may need to have follow-up care by a specialist

Other Types of Healthcare

Telemedicine (also known as: _telehealth, e-health, m-health [mobile health]_)

Telemedicine is a rapidly growing brand of healthcare that utilizes many facets of technology. Its purpose is to promote health through the electronic exchange of medical information. This communication can occur between hospitals, home health agencies, medical and specialty offices, and patient homes.

According to the American Telemedicine Association (ATA), "_Telemedicine is the remote delivery of healthcare services and clinical information using telecommunications technology._" This technology is used to exchange medical information from one site to another through the use of Internet, wireless, satellite, and telephone media. The devices commonly used to do this are two-way video, email, computers, and smart phones. The transferable information can include: patient office visits via video conferencing, electronic transmission of photos and x-ray pictures, and remote monitoring of health information. _Two-way video conferencing_, an online medical visit, can be done from a medical facility or from the home. The technology can be managed with the help of healthcare personnel, such as a visiting nurse, or independently by the patient.

As of this writing, healthcare services using Telemedicine include:

- online support groups
- electronic communication with providers
- electronic health records
- the transmission of home health monitoring, such as blood pressure, blood sugar, or symptoms
- remote monitoring of heart pacemakers

A current search of the pros and cons of Telemedicine reveals the following:

Pros:

- Convenience
- Less time spent in waiting rooms
- Cost-efficient
- Expedited transmission of MRI and x-ray films
- Privacy assurance: complies with HIPAA Privacy and Patient Confidentiality rules
- Extended specialist and referring physician access, including those professionals requested for a second opinion
- Increased patient/provider communication
- More access to specialty practices
- Visits can be done in the home
- Review of x-rays by a Radiologist at any time of the day or night
- Increased rural access

Cons:

- Electronic glitches
- Technical training: All staff, medical and non-medical, are required to be trained on how to use the technology according to their specific departmental needs

- Resistance to new and changing technology
- Limited or inadequate exam: There is a decreased ability for the provider to observe non-verbal body language and no ability to personally touch or feel the problem area. To some patients, this can feel like a depersonalized experience
- Reduced continuity of care: A patient's primary care provider may not have access to the Telemedicine health record, resulting in an incomplete medical history. Also, when seen by different Telemedicine providers, the patient may have to review their past medical history *with each new provider*, if that provider does not have access to their current medical record
- Fewer in-person (face-to-face) consultations
- Rules regarding healthcare laws, licensing and credentials, reimbursement policies, and privacy protection vary from state to state. While Telemedicine complies with the HIPAA privacy act, keeping up with this fast-growing industry can be a struggle
- Informed Consent: you must sign a consent stating that you understand the advantages and potential concerns associated with medical treatments via Telemedicine

Concierge Medicine (also known as: *boutique medicine, retainer-based medicine, direct care*)

Concierge Medicine, another clinic option, is a form of healthcare in which the patient pays an annual fee of hundreds to thousands of dollars (a *retainer*) to the clinic practice in return for more personalized services. This may include quicker access to the provider with shorter wait times, a longer time given during an office visit, access to the provider any time of day or night, personal coordination of care with specialists, home visits, and access to the provider's cellphone number and email. While there are similarities among all the types of concierge medicine, they can vary widely in their structure, payment requirements, and form of operation.

Concierge care is *not* a replacement for health insurance. While wellness visits and primary care are typically covered under the plan, the retainer does not cover any necessary out-of-office visits to specialists, Urgent Care or Emergency Room visits, surgery, and high-tech diagnostic testing, such as MRI and CT. Moreover, the retainer is not reimbursed by private health insurance or Medicare, although some concierge practices may bill the insurance company for some of the services provided. You may choose to have concierge care for your primary care, *and* then have insurance for healthcare that is outside of the concierge practice.

If you are considering concierge care, review the following questions to make a determination as to whether this medical option is right for you:

- Do they offer after-hours care?
- Does the clinic take insurance, and will they file claims for you?
- What is the fee and what services are included in that fee?
- What preventive care is covered?
- Will the provider admit you to the hospital if it is necessary, or will you be seen by the hospitalist? (A specialist who gives care to a hospitalized patient only)
- Do they schedule same-day appointments?
- Who do you contact for questions and how?
- Will they coordinate your care with your specialists (who lie outside of the concierge care)?
- Do they make house calls?
- Will they accept HSA (health savings account) debit cards issued by your insurance company? Likewise, will your HSA cover the fees for this type of practice?

Special Accident/Injury Situations

There are certain medical circumstances that require you to seek healthcare in a different way.

If an injury occurs while you are at work, contact your supervisor or the Human Resources department for instructions. *Workers Compensation*, also known as *workman's comp*, is a state-mandated insurance program that provides wage replacement and medical benefits to employees who suffer job-related injuries and illnesses. Review your policy manual or meet with the Human Resource's department for any questions regarding Workers Compensation.

If an injury occurs as a result of a motor vehicle accident (whether or not it is your fault), tell the medical reception desk when you are checking in. Auto insurance must *first* be considered for payment before filing with your health insurance company. If you are involved in a non-life threatening accident, contact your insurance agent as soon as possible to see what steps you need to take.

CHAPTER 3

All About Appointments
(Not more Paperwork!)

Once you decide on the name of your desired provider or a group of providers, it is time to think about actually making an appointment.

If you are already established with the provider you want to see, scheduling the appointment can be relatively painless. The clinic already has most of the needed information, and you are familiar with the scheduling process.

However, if you are scheduling an appointment with a new provider, you may find it a little frightening. That's normal. Know that regardless of why you are seeking healthcare, the receptionist will be asking you specific questions. Keep in mind that the front office staff of any medical clinic are the gate keepers, and they have been instructed by their supervisors and providers on how to do their job. *Help them find out what they need to know.*

Anticipating what the clinic receptionist will ask you prior to calling for the appointment will help lessen any pressure you may be feeling. So before you actually call for the appointment, you may want to seat yourself at a table. Place in front of you a pen and a piece of paper, your calendar (which includes already scheduled events and appointments), and your insurance card (if you have one).

If you are scheduling an appointment following a visit to the Urgent Care or Emergency Room, have your discharge paperwork handy. Highlight the specific provider's name, the phone number, the diagnosis, or any other particulars that may be helpful to the receptionist before you call.

Then pick up the phone.

Making the Call

Don't be surprised if, after dialing, you hear a recorded message instructing you to push a certain number, depending on the need. If you miss the number for a specific provider or to schedule the appointment, keep listening until the end of the recording. There will usually be instructions so that you can repeat the options.

Once you have the scheduling receptionist on the line, all the information you have in front of you will come into play. Begin by giving your name and the provider's name you wish to make an appointment with. If you don't have a specific provider name, ask for a provider who is accepting new patients and/or who is first available. The receptionist will take it from there. They may ask:

- If you have seen this provider, or have you been a patient at this practice before
- What the problem is
- If you have been referred by another provider, and who that provider is (for example, "Were you referred by a primary care provider, a specialist, Urgent Care, or the Emergency Room?")
- Which Urgent Care, Emergency Room, or hospital you were at, and the date you were there
- If you have insurance, and if so, the name of the insurance company. You may have to give them your group number and member ID, two pieces of information usually found on the front of insurance cards. If you don't have insurance, let them know, and be sure to ask what the self-pay policy is

When you are on the phone scheduling your appointment, you may find it is tricky to find a time that works for both parties. Please don't take it personally if you find out you are not going to be seen in the near future. In many busy medical clinics, it is not uncommon for new patients to have to wait two to three months for their first office visit. (If you are already established with the requested provider, it usually will be easier to get an earlier appointment.). Many clinics will allot a greater amount of time for new patient visits, which allows the patient and provider time to get to know each other.

If you need to get in within the month and are considered a new patient, many times there will be little flexibility, particularly with specialists. My advice is to take the first available appointment that is offered (assuming you are available at that time, and if not, try to make yourself available). Many times specialists will "work in" patients into an already full schedule.

If you absolutely cannot make the offered appointment, talk with the receptionist about other available times. If you have been told by your provider to schedule an appointment on a specific date or during a specific time frame, tell the receptionist. They will do what they can to accommodate you.

If you can't get an appointment as early as desired, ask if the clinic keeps a list of patients to call if there are any cancellations, and if so, ask to be added to it. If a list is not available, ask the receptionist if you can call periodically to see if there have been any cancellations.

If you have the option of choosing an appointment time, consider selecting an early morning or early afternoon appointment, if possible. The chance of a provider running behind increases with each patient visit. So, you are less likely to have to wait if you are the first appointment of the day, or the first appointment after the office breaks for lunch.

If you are very sick and need to see a provider as soon as possible, tell the receptionist this when you call to schedule your appointment. They will do everything they can to get you in quickly. If this is not option, the receptionist may refer you to the Urgent Care or Emergency Room. Again, establishing with a provider before it is needed saves you time and energy.

If you call to schedule an appointment with your provider and they are not available, you may be asked if you would like to see a different provider. (This may be a physician, nurse practitioner, or physician's assistant.) Or, you may be given the option to wait until your provider is available.

Most clinics provide coverage for when a provider is unavailable, but this is not always the case. When establishing with a provider, it may be helpful to ask what happens when the provider is unavailable and you need to be seen.

When calling to schedule an appointment with a provider, especially if you have been seen before, the receptionist will ask you about the reason for the visit. If you would like extra things to be done, in addition to the main reason for the visit, tell the receptionist at this time. This could include services such as: a flu shot, request for a specific blood test, and/or filling out of forms, such as for insurance, a handicapped/disability license plate or placard, the Family Medical Leave Act, or work-related. Know that some medical clinics will charge a fee to fill out the paperwork, which may not be covered by your insurance.

If at all possible, arrive to your appointment at least fifteen minutes before the scheduled time. Know that the process of checking in, obtaining your vital signs, and having you ready for the provider takes time. Arriving at your scheduled appointment time or later can cause the clinic staff to run behind, along with all the patients that follow you.

If you make an appointment but are unable to keep it, always notify the office you aren't coming, even if it is at the last minute. This gives you the opportunity to reschedule your appointment. The clinic is then able to schedule another patient into your slot, and they'll know not to wait for you.

Many medical clinics will contact you to remind you of an upcoming office visit. Know that some clinics will charge you for an office visit if you do not call and do not show up to your scheduled appointment. Other clinics will still charge you a fee if you cancel within a twenty-four-hour window of the appointment time.

If at all possible, arrive to your appointment at least fifteen minutes before the scheduled time. Know that the process of checking in, obtaining your vital signs, and having you ready for the provider takes time. Arriving at your scheduled appointment time or later can cause the clinic staff to run behind, along with all the patients that follow you.

There are clinics that will discharge you from the clinic practice when you do not call and do not show up to a certain number of appointments. Realize health clinics count on paid office visits to support their business. When you can't keep your appointment and don't call, the clinic does not have the chance to fill that appointment time with another patient, resulting in potential loss of income.

When you are establishing yourself as a patient with any new provider, there will be a number of questions and a certain amount of paperwork you can expect. The requested information typically includes demographic information (name, address, phone number, date of birth, etc.), insurance information, past medical history (diagnoses, surgeries, childbirth history), family history, history of the current illness, and emergency contacts. All of this information helps the medical clinic to get to know you and to provide you with quality care. It is important, that once established, you report any changes in your contact information at your next visit, especially your phone number, in the event the clinic has to contact you.

The health clinic may obtain all the necessary information from you by the following ways, depending on the type of system used by that particular clinic:

- The receptionist obtains some of the information over the phone during your initial call, with the rest gathered in person when you first arrive and check in with the receptionist
- You fill out the information forms when you first arrive at the clinic. If so, plan to come fifteen to thirty minutes early to complete the paperwork. The receptionist may specifically advise you on how early to come. The paperwork may request some of the information listed above

- If you think there will be too many forms to fill out at one time and/or you have a disability which prevents you from filing out the new patient paperwork quickly, you can ask to pick up the necessary forms, fill them out at home, and bring them back to the receptionist at your scheduled appointment time. This option allows you time, and you will not feel rushed to read the material and fill in all the blanks. Plus, it also gives you the opportunity to look up any information you don't remember or have at the ready
- The provider may mail the forms or email you forms to download onto your computer, allowing you to fill them out at home before the appointment
- The referring medical provider or facility will forward the necessary information via fax, mail, or electronically to your provider
- From your Electronic Health Record (EHR). (Electronic Health Records will be discussed later in this chapter)
- The receptionist may hand you a tablet or small electronic device for you to enter your information. Or, you may be asked to sit at a desktop computer and enter your information in. If you are uncomfortable using any of the electronic devices offered, do not feel embarrassed to ask the receptionist for assistance or to see if paper forms are available

Physician-Patient Arbitration Agreement

You may or may not have noticed that one of the forms you *might* have been asked to sign is a Physician-Patient Arbitration Agreement. In this contract, you, the patient, agree to bring any medical malpractice claims you may have against your healthcare provider to *arbitration*, in place of filing a *medical malpractice lawsuit* in court.

Arbitration is a method of resolving medical malpractice disputes outside of court. It utilizes independent third-party *arbitrators* on both sides of the table to review evidence, listen to the parties, and then make a decision. There is no judge or jury. The arbitrators act as both.

In a *medical malpractice lawsuit*, the medical malpractice claim is disputed in a court of law before a judge and jury.

Should you be asked to sign this form and do not want to, ask the receptionist if you have the option not to. And if you choose not to sign it, ask if you can still see your preferred provider. Medical clinics have the option to refuse services to you if you refuse to sign the agreement.

Notice that some agreements include a retroactive clause, meaning the agreement covers not only services after the date signed, but also services given to you by that provider/clinic *before* it was signed.

There may also be a clause allowing you to revoke the agreement if your request is submitted to the clinic/provider within a certain amount of time after signing.

Carefully review your health insurance policy. Some health insurance plan agreements contain language in which the patient agrees beforehand that any medical malpractice claim will be heard by an arbitrator and not in court.

If you are considering signing an Arbitration Agreement or have already signed one, and have questions or concerns about what it all means, consult with a medical malpractice attorney. They are the experts, and they will know how to advise you.

Arriving for the Appointment

If there is more than one concern you wish to discuss with your provider at your appointment, be sure to make a list *before* coming to your appointment. This will help you to remember what you want to talk about during your visit. Be sure to place your most important two or three issues *at the top of this list,* so that there is enough time to cover what is of most concern to you when your healthcare provider sees you. Also, having this piece of paper handy at your visit gives you a place to write down the provider's answers and any instructions you receive.

When you arrive at the office or clinic, arrive expecting to wait. So it's smart to bring something with you to do, especially if you are going to have children accompanying you - for any time spent in the waiting room. Wear clothing that is loose-fitting and comfortable. Bring a snack and something to drink, if you feel this may be necessary for your health.

Right as you are about to enter the office or clinic, observe whether there are separate entrances or waiting rooms for sick and well patients. If so, choose that which is appropriate for your needs at this particular visit. You likely will discover that some pediatricians have separate waiting rooms for sick and healthy children. If yours does not, and you or your children may have something contagious, sit away from other patients if at all possible.

When you first walk into the clinic or office, check in at the receptionist's window. Give them your name. Confirm your appointment time and the provider you will be seeing. You may be asked to sign your name on a sign-in sheet.

Expect to fill out and/or sign some type of paperwork with each and every office visit. While much can be done electronically, there is still a dependence on paper. Symptoms of your illness, review of contact information, and signatures may be required. As healthcare is in a constant state of change, so is the required documentation. Getting upset with the receptionist because they give you another form to sign does no good. They are only doing their job.

Always bring an identification card (ID), such as your driver's license or passport, and your insurance card, if you have one. Even if you have been to your provider's clinic several times, there is always a chance the receptionist may need a copy. Many health clinics are now asking to take a photo of you for their *electronic health record (EHR)*.

What is an EHR? Something that has radically changed the face of healthcare.

Understanding the Electronic Health Record (EHR; *also known as an Electronic Medical Record – EMR*)

An *Electronic Health Record (EHR)* is:

> ...an electronic version of a patient's medical history, that is maintained by the provider over time, and may include all of the key administrative clinical data relevant to that person's care under a particular provider, including demographics, progress notes, problems, medications, vital signs, past medical history, immunizations, laboratory data and radiology reports. The EHR automates access to information and has the potential to streamline the clinician's workflow. The EHR also has the ability to support other care-related activities directly or indirectly through various interfaces, including evidence-based decision support, quality management, and outcomes reporting. - Centers for Medicare and Medicaid Services (CMMS)

Basically, the EHR has taken the place of a paper chart of your medical history. Your health information may now be in an electronic chart that can be found in the computer.

There are many advantages of an EHR:

- Includes all patient-related information
- Can be updated at any time by your provider
- Information can be found quickly and brought up by the medical staff
- Can be viewed by other consulting providers

- Allows for quicker and more efficient data-gathering and number analysis
- Monitors activity in the patient's health after changes in medications, procedures, diet, or activity
- Flags the provider when the patient is due for follow-up, such as with wellness physicals, vaccines, lab tests, and other procedures
- Encourages communication between the patient and their provider
- Reduces the risk of medical errors. For example, if a new medication is added to a list of medications, the EHR can identify possible drug interactions between them. Also, if the patient sees multiple providers within a healthcare system, all may see any medication changes initiated by one or more providers. This can, as a result, influence a provider's decision to start or stop a medication
- Improves the accuracy and clarity of medical records, such as having to read illegible handwriting
- Reduces healthcare costs by improving the quality of healthcare. This is accomplished by making the health information readily available, reducing repeat testing, and reducing delays in treatment
- Can assist in the billing and coding process, which is necessary for the payment (reimbursement) of provider services from insurance companies

Yet while medicine recognizes the benefits of computers, it is constantly aware of the risks. There are drawbacks, too:

- Limits the use of the EHR by those who do not have access to a computer, or who do not have the knowledge to use a computer
- While each healthcare system will utilize a certain brand of EHR throughout its organization, there is no guarantee the competing healthcare system will use the same one. This makes it harder for opposing systems to share your health record electronically, if it is medically necessary
- Learning how to correctly use the EHR will take time for both provider and patient, especially for those who are used to a paper chart or who have had little computer experience
- The EHR may need to be looked at and added to by nearly every person in the clinic: reception, lab/x-ray, medical records, medical assistants, and providers, for example. So your EHR can be seen by unauthorized eyes (as is also the case with paper charts)

- There is a risk of unauthorized access to your protected health information by hackers and by theft of electronic devices containing health information

The Health Insurance Portability and Accountability Act of 1996 (HIPAA) specifically addresses this subject:

> The HIPAA Privacy Rule establishes national standards to protect individuals' medical records and other personal health information and applies to health plans, healthcare clearinghouses, and those healthcare providers that conduct certain healthcare transactions electronically. The Rule requires appropriate safeguards to protect the privacy of personal health information, and sets limits and conditions on the uses and disclosures that may be made of such information without patient authorization. The Rule also gives patients' rights over their health information, including rights to examine and obtain a copy of their health records, and to request corrections. - U.S. Department of Health and Human Services

Financial penalties for civil offenses range from $100 to $50,000, per offense, for unauthorized individuals who look at your electronic or paper health record, with an annual maximum of $1.5 million. In addition, if the individual works within the healthcare system, they risk losing their job as a result. Criminal offenses, in which health information is gained under false pretense or used for personal gain or malicious harm, can result in fines up to $250,000 and up to ten years in prison.

At a medical visit, some of the initial paperwork you will receive or be offered teaches you about HIPAA. More information on HIPAA can be found at the U.S. Department of Health and Human Service's website: www.hhs.gov/ocr/privacy/hipaa/understanding/consumers/index.html.

As an added reassurance, healthcare systems and EHR businesses work to protect patient confidentiality by continually updating firewall and security programs, installing and maintaining anti-virus software, utilizing strong password requirements and screen saver locks, and by requiring annual employee HIPAA training.

Understanding the Personal Health Record (PHR)

In comparison to an Electronic Health Record (EHR), a *Personal Health Record (PHR)* is a web-based personal health record of *your* health, available to you on *your* computer or device. It is information about *your* health, *and is put together and maintained by you.* This information may include your demographic information, such as age, birthdate, address, marital status, and occupation, medical history, clinic progress notes, and test results.

With a PHR, you have control over how the health information is obtained, used, and made public. Yet it is important to recall that PHRs are separate from, and do not replace, the legal record of any healthcare provider. PHRs are not considered legal health records, thus are not covered by HIPAA. (The EHR *is* a legal record and *is* covered by HIPAA.)

Many, but not all, healthcare EHR systems include a PHR option for you. This means once you enroll yourself with your healthcare system's EHR, you may be given the option to set up a PHR. When you do this, you are able to electronically communicate with your provider through your PHR. Also, your health information, such as diagnoses and test results, will be added as they occur. Know that should you leave this healthcare system, you may or may not have access to your PHR, which is attached to your EHR.

Whether you have a Personal Health Record with your healthcare system or one independent of it, you will now have access to your medical record wherever you go. You may have the option to transfer information directly from your EHR. Or, you can scan and download documents into the desired files of your PHR. You can print copies of your medical information, if needed. You can track what testing you've had done, when you had it done, and what the results were. You can keep in one place a history of your previous hospitalizations and procedures.

As with the EHR, there is the risk of unlawful online access with a PHR. Security is maintained the same as with the EHR and is performed by each individual company. The EHR and PHR may be owned by the same company and use the same security systems.

Waiting...

When checking in - especially for the first time - consider asking the receptionist what to do if you have a medical question after clinic hours. The receptionist can explain the procedures for leaving phones messages for non-urgent concerns, such as a medication refill or question, and what to do if you experience an urgent medical problem.

Once you have handled anything that the receptionist has requested of you, settle yourself down to wait. *Patiently.* Remain considerate of others in the waiting room, especially when talking on the phone or playing loud video games.

Should you find that thirty minutes has passed and you are still waiting, ask the receptionist how much longer they anticipate your wait will be. Continue to do so at fifteen to thirty minute intervals. As you will see in the following chapter, there are many reasons medical visits run late. If time allows, continue to wait. If not, speak with the receptionist. Tell them you are unable to wait any longer and reschedule your appointment, knowing the process may be repeated on your return visit.

CHAPTER 4

The Office Visit

(A patient may have only one provider, but the provider has many patients)

Your wait is over. You finally make it past the front desk. The assistant calls out your name and escorts you through the waiting room door.

What happens now?

Many times, the medical assistant will weigh you on a scale in the corridor before you enter the examination room. They may also measure your height and determine your body-mass index (BMI = a measure of body fat based on your height and weight).

Once you are seated in the exam room, the assistant may or may not obtain your vital signs, such as blood pressure, temperature, and pulse. They will ask you a few questions about your health, and write the answers down on the chart or enter the information into the computer. At this time, tell the assistant your most important health concerns, so they may document them for the provider to see before they enter the room. This gives the provider a chance to formulate questions and a tentative plan of care. Those assisting you for the provider may include:

- Registered Nurse (RN)
  Education:
  > Diploma in Nursing (a hospital-based nursing program): two to three years of education
  > > *Mary Smith, RN*
  > Associate Degree in Nursing (ADN); Associate of Science in Nursing (ASN); Associate of Applied Science in Nursing (AAS): two to three years of education

Mary Smith, ADN, RN,
Mary Smith, ASN, RN
Mary Smith, AAS, RN
Bachelor of Science in Nursing (BSN): four years of education
Mary Smith, BSN, RN
Certification: The National Council of State Boards of Nursing:
National Council Licensure Examination (NCLEX)

- <u>Licensed Practical Nurse (LPN)</u>; <u>Licensed Vocational Nurse (LVN)</u>
Education: one to two years
Mary Smith, LPN
Mary Smith, LVN
Certification: The National Council of State Boards of Nursing:
National Council Licensure Examination Practical Nurse (NCLEX-PN)

- <u>Certified Medical Assistant (CMA)</u>
Education:
Certificate or Diploma: one year
Associate degree: two years
Certification: It is not required for medical assistants to be certified or registered but may be recommended or required in some medical practices.
American Association of Medical Assistants certification examination
Mary Smith, CMA (certified medical assistant)
The American Registry of Medical Assistants
Mary Smith, RMA (registered medical assistant)

If the medical office visit requires that you undress, the assistant will have laid out a gown and sheet on the table that will most likely be disposable. Disposable products cost less and are easier to supply (versus sending linens to the laundry). The assistant will ask you to undress and then exit the room so you have privacy while changing.

Anytime a male provider is to examine a female patient's reproductive parts (breasts or genital area), a female or male medical professional chaperone (witness) can be requested to be in the room. Likewise, if a female provider must examine a male patient's genitals, a female or male medical professional chaperone can be requested. This is to ensure that no inappropriate physical contact or verbal communication takes place between the provider and the patient while the patient is undressed. Some clinics require a chaperone to be present while others do not. If you know that you will need to be undressed and do not want to be seen by the opposite sex, please make this request known when you are scheduling your appointment so arrangements can be made.

The medical staff will have you get yourself ready before the provider arrives to save on time. The scheduling receptionist has allotted each patient a certain amount of time to be seen by the provider. This allows the office to be efficient and to stay on schedule. So it is likely that the office has several patients waiting in their respective rooms at one time.

For your wait, have a coat or blanket handy in case you get chilly. Here, too, you might want to bring something to do in case the wait proves long.

The Interaction With Your Provider

When your provider enters the room and sees you, the patient, they want to see all of you - how you walk and talk, the way you get up onto the exam table, and your general appearance. Even if you are not able to care for yourself, your provider still wants to make eye contact with you and communicate through talk and touch.

Many providers have the option to *precept* students who are in school to obtain the same degree as the provider. This means the student is allowed to follow the provider (*preceptor*) when seeing patients. There may be times when the student will evaluate the patient first, then discuss their findings with the provider, followed by both reviewing the plan of care with the patient. The provider instructs the student on patient care specific to their area of study. These students may include medical students, Interns and Residents, and physician assistant and nurse practitioner students. Prior to being allowed to precept with a provider, the student's educational institution must have a contract with the healthcare center. Also, the student must sign a Confidentiality Agreement stating they will not discuss patients' healthcare outside of the learning arena. So if there is a student in the room with you and your provider, know that this is a teaching situation and be assured that your confidentiality is secure. If you do not want to be interviewed and/or examined by a student or Resident physician, please tell the assistant or provider. You have the option to decline this service.

As you are being seen, be sure to discuss your most important concerns first (referring to your list if need be). When you bring these issues up, be wary of what is a question or worry, and what a complaint is. In most cases, your provider will be able to easily answer any direct questions or worries. However, complaints can take on a life of their own. So if you are unhappy about something, calmly state the concern and ask if there's anything to be done about it. If so, your provider will tell you. If not, your provider will assist you with your concern the best that they can. And then it is necessary to move on.

Recognize that your provider sees many patients a day, all of whom have many questions and concerns of their own. The provider wants to help out each individual patient and address all concerns but doing so is not always feasible. While the provider's goal is to take care of all a patient's healthcare needs in one visit, it may not be possible when there is a limited amount of time, a long list of concerns, and a schedule full of patients. If time runs short and you cannot cover every item on your list, re-schedule a follow-up visit to address additional concerns.

During the office visit, there may be an "assistant" using the computer while the provider talks to you and examines you. Many offices are using *"scribes"*, an assistant who enters information into the computer. This allows your provider to ask questions and perform the examination while dictating to the scribe, who enters the information into the computer. Scribes can save the provider time and increase the efficiency of the medical practice. The provider then can review the notes later and make any necessary changes.

There are certain types of providers that must be on-call, meaning they must be available to perform a medical service at a moment's notice. This would include an obstetrician, who delivers babies, and a surgeon, who performs emergency surgery. If your provider is called away during office hours for an emergency, the receptionist should inform all waiting patients what has happened. They may give you the option to wait, be seen by a different provider, or reschedule your appointment. They may also be able to give you an estimate of time in which they anticipate the provider's return.

Should Family Members Be at the Appointment With You?

Bringing a family member or loved one with you to your appointment can be helpful. They may be able to offer information related to your health - information you may have forgotten, or were not even aware of. They also can take notes and/or recall parts of the visit you may not be able to remember later on. There are times, though, when a family member or loved one may interfere with the relationship between you and your provider.

Having your family member or loved one offer specific pieces of information and calmly discuss your health with your permission can be helpful. Demanding certain tests be run on you, arguing about the results you are receiving, interrupting the exchange of information with your provider, and questioning the actions of the provider is not helpful.

When your provider is talking directly to you, the patient, it is not appropriate for your family member or loved one to respond. The time for your family member or loved one to share information is when the provider addresses them, when the provider has finished talking with you, or before the provider begins his exam. (If the provider is made aware of the health concern prior to starting the exam, they can easily include that information in their examination). So in advance, encourage family members and loved ones not to interrupt you while you are answering the provider's question. If there is something that they feel needs to be added, have them wait until you are finished with the dialogue. The family member or loved one can also tell the medical assistant their concerns when they first are seated in the room. The provider will then be aware of the concern prior to entering the room.

If your family member or loved one wants to tell your provider about a concern they have about you before or after your visit, they are free to call your provider's office and speak with your provider's nurse. This can be a helpful thing to do, especially for those situations when the family member or loved one wishes to share information with your provider that will benefit your health, but do not want to embarrass you in the process. For example, if you are elderly and experiencing poor judgment or reflex skills, and are continuing to drive, your family is able to call your provider's nurse and explain what is going on. At your next medical visit, after examining you, your provider can voice their concern and recommend you not drive any longer. You may be more inclined to follow the instructions of your provider than the requests of your family or loved ones. Because of privacy rules, the nurse can take a loved one's message or information, but can't give them any information in return unless you have signed the privacy papers stating it is okay to do so.

Understanding What's Happening

Once the provider has addressed your main concerns and has completed the exam, there may be changes made to your old prescription, prescriptions given for new medications, further tests to be run on you, recommendations about undergoing a procedure, and/or referrals to other providers. Regardless of whether these changes are minor adjustments or significant, it is very important for you to have a basic understanding of why they are being made.

If something was brought up that you do not understand, *ask the provider before they walk out the door*. You may not get another chance to ask and/or may forget by the next visit.

Should the provider walk out before you can get the explanation, ask the medical assistant your question should they come back in to discharge you, or when checking out. If they do not know the answer, they should be able to find out before you leave. Consider making some notes right after the visit to remember what was said, and write down any questions you come up with later for the next visit.

If you are older and have trouble with hearing, communicating, or remembering what was said, be sure a companion is present to make notes and help ask and/or answer questions. Or, consider using your cell phone to make notes. Most contain a recorder as well as a note-taking app, which may be helpful in remembering your discharge instructions. Or, use your phone to text or email yourself a series of notes.

When a test has been ordered, it's important to know where it can be done. Some offices have lab and x-ray facilities in their building, while other offices require you to go elsewhere. "*Diagnostic centers*" contain a variety of testing services, including lab, x-ray, mammogram, bone mineral density, CT, MRI, and ultrasound. You will receive a piece of paper with the name of the test on it. Sometimes, the name and the address of the diagnostic center or testing facility will also be on it. This is the order that is to be given to the facility. If you are unsure on where to go or how to schedule the test, review the matter with the medical assistant or the receptionist. If you have insurance, make sure the diagnostic center is in-network. If you don't have insurance, you can price-shop by calling the different diagnostic centers to compare pricing.

If you are to have a test that requires you to be fasting, make a note of the specific instructions on the appointment card, the order sheet, your phone, or some place that causes you to remember. Fasting guidelines vary among tests. Some may require you have an empty stomach while others will allow water or black coffee.

If you are being referred to another provider or specialist, your provider will most likely refer you to someone who is in-network (as they will typically be in the same healthcare system). It does not hurt to confirm that this is so. You may receive a piece of paper with the new consulting provider's name, address, contact information, and referring diagnosis. In most cases, it will be your responsibility to schedule this appointment. If the new provider is in the same healthcare system, they may receive the referral and your information electronically through your electronic health record (EHR). So when you call to schedule, it is likely they will have most everything they need.

Once your visit with your provider is complete, you will be asked to stop at the check-out desk before leaving. The provider will indicate to you and/or the staff as to when you are to be seen again. Please remember that your provider has an ethical and legal responsibility to monitor your health. If the provider requests that you come back sooner than you feel necessary, please schedule back as they have requested. It is in your health's best interest to follow the provider's instructions.

It is at this time (when you are at the check-out desk) that any appropriate payment is made. If there is a co-pay, this is when you should pay it. If you have no insurance and payment wasn't made before the office visit, this is when you should pay it or make arrangements to do so.

It is important to keep track of all your healthcare receipts in the event of a billing discrepancy. You may not receive some medical bills until weeks, or sometimes months, after the office visit. Keep the bill and receipt of payment together for quick reference, should it be necessary. If you have insurance, include your Explanation of Benefits (EOB) form with this paperwork.

The Billing Process

For those with insurance, the billing process is quite intricate. And because of the differences between insurance plans, it is impractical to have an in depth discussion of how it all works. Therefore, I will give you an overview of the medical insurance billing process.

As we reviewed in Chapter 2, a Managed Care Organization (MCO) is an organization that combines the functions of health insurance, delivery of care, and administration into one package. MCO is an umbrella term for health plans that provide healthcare in return for a predetermined monthly fee and coordinate care through a defined network of physicians and hospitals.

MCOs contract directly with *healthcare providers and healthcare systems* - the plan's *network* - to provide care for a plan's members at a reduced cost. By providing a wide variety of quality healthcare services to enrolled workers, they are able to keep medical costs down. How much of your care your plan will pay for depends on your insurance company and the network's rules. Plans that limit your choices usually cost less. More flexible plans probably cost more.

As a general rule: The higher your deductible = the lower your premium = the more you will pay out-of-pocket for healthcare services (to meet your deductible). The lower your deductible = the higher your premium = the less you will pay out of pocket to meet your deductible (but you will be paying more in premiums).

In review, the four major types of managed care plans are:

- *Health Maintenance Organizations (HMO)*: You must choose a primary care provider (PCP), and the insurance company usually only pays for care *within the network*
- *Preferred Provider Organizations (PPO)*: You can visit any in-network health-care provider without obtaining a referral from your PCP. Staying inside the network costs you, as a member, less. You may seek healthcare outside of the network without a referral, but this costs more
- *Point of Service (POS)*: You must choose a PCP. If the PCP refers you to a specialist in the network, your costs will be lower. If you choose to see a provider outside of the network, your costs will be higher
- *Exclusive Provider Organizations (EPO)*: You must use providers from a specific network. You won't need to choose a primary care provider, and you don't need referrals to see a specialist. There is no coverage for care received outside of the network, except in cases of emergency

And now a review of basic insurance terms:

- *Deductible*: A fixed dollar amount that an insured person pays before the insurance company starts to make payments for covered medical services. The amount you pay out-of-pocket and how much of that money your insurance company applies toward your deductible may vary if services are received from an approved (in-network) provider versus an out-of-network provider. Some in-network services may be covered by your insurance company before you have met your deductible. The deductible benefit period is typically for one year
- *Co-insurance*: the percentage of money you pay for each healthcare service, office visit, or prescription after your deductible has been paid
- *Co-pay* (co-payment): the fixed amount you pay for each healthcare service provided, such as for an office visit or a prescription
- *Premium*: the fee you agree to pay for coverage of medical benefits in a defined period of time. For example, every two weeks your employer deducts the insurance premium from your paycheck
- *In-Network*: a group of physicians, hospitals, and other healthcare providers that agree to provide medical services at pre-negotiated rates with your insurance company

- *Maximum out-of-pocket:* the most you will have to pay for covered medical expenses in a plan year. The maximum is reached through deductible, coinsurance, and out-of-pocket contributions. Once you have paid the maximum out-of-pocket, your insurance plan begins to pay 100 percent of *covered* medical expenses for the remainder of the plan year
- *Explanation of Benefits (EOB):* statement from your insurance company that summarizes the billed charges from all the providers and medical facilities, payments made by your insurance company, prescription payments, and the estimate of what is owed by you. (Keep in mind this is just a summary and not the actual bill)

It is important for patients with insurance to know what their *deductible, co-insurance percentage,* and *maximum out-of-pocket* is. All of these numbers play a role in a health insurance claim.

Example Scenario: *These numbers will vary based on your individual plan.*

For the last five years, you have been paying a monthly insurance *premium* of $400. You can see this deduction on your pay stub. You are now experiencing a serious illness and have accumulated $50,000 in medical expenses.

Your *deductible* is $5,000.

Your *co-insurance* is 20 percent.

Your *maximum out-of-pocket* is $6,000.

1. You are responsible for the first $5,000 (deductible)
2. After you pay your $5,000, you are responsible for the 20 percent *co-insurance* until you reach your *maximum out-of-pocket* of $6,000.
   - $50,000 (expenses) - $5,000 (deductible paid by you) = $45,000
   - $45,000 x 20 percent ($45,000 x 0.2; co-insurance) = $9,000
   - Because your maximum out-of-pocket cost is $6,000, and you have already paid the $5,000 deductible, you will pay $1,000 co-insurance.
3. Your insurance company may then pay 100 percent of the *allowed amount for covered services.* They will take into consideration if the medical care provided is within your insurance network, if it is out-of-network, and the UCR (what is usual, customary, and reasonable) rate. You may receive a bill for the amount not covered by your insurance company. *Bear in mind, at the beginning of each contract year, your out-of-pocket fees go back to the original amount.*

The next question in your mind is probably where the figure of $50,000 in medical expenses comes from. This number is a result of an even more complicated process called *Coding and Billing*.

Coding and Billing

Coding and Billing are two closely related components of the insurance reimbursement cycle, which ensures that healthcare providers and facilities are paid for their services. Coders and Billers can be trained to do both jobs and are often located in the same office.

Medical coding is the conversion of healthcare diagnoses, procedures, medical services, and equipment into universal medical alpha-numeric codes (contain letters and numbers). There is a specific corresponding code for *every* diagnosis, injury, medical procedure, and type of office visit. For example, there are many considerations that go into coding an office visit, such as:

1. Are you a new or established patient?
2. The type of visit you had: Is it a wellness check-up or a sick visit?
3. How sick you are: How many diagnoses do you have?
4. The length of time the provider spends with you
5. The number of exams the provider performs: How much of your body did the provider examine?

What is the difference between a wellness or preventive exam and a physical or sick visit?

A *Physical Exam* is the thorough examination of the body to determine if there is or is not a physical problem. During this type of visit, a previously identified medical problem (e.g., high blood pressure and diabetes) can also be monitored and illnesses can be evaluated (*sick visit*). This exam usually includes:

- Looking at the body (inspection)
- Feeling the body with fingers or hands (palpation)
- Listening to the body's sounds (auscultation)
- Producing sounds, usually by tapping on areas of the body (percussion)

A *Wellness Exam* is used to develop or update your personal *preventive* health plan. This visit includes:

- A health risk assessment (questions you answer about your health)
- A review of your medical and family medical history
- Developing or updating a list of your current providers and prescriptions
- Documenting your height, weight, blood pressure and other routine measurements
- Looking for signs of memory loss or dementia
- Personalized health advice just for you
- A list of risk factors and treatment options for you
- Receiving recommended vaccines
- A screening schedule (like a checklist) for the preventive services recommended for you, such as a mammogram

Many times a provider will combine a physical exam with a wellness visit, which can save you time and money. And, it is not uncommon for these terms to be used interchangeably, along with other regional variations. The problem comes when it's time to *code* the visit for insurance purposes.

When your in-network provider strictly uses a *screening (preventive)* code, this type of visit may be covered by your insurance company, without cost to you, as it falls under "Preventive Health".

Should your provider use a *diagnosis* code, meaning a health problem has been identified and given a diagnosis (e.g., high blood or bronchitis), your insurance plan may require you to pay your co-pay, or your deductible may need to be met, before the insurance company begins making payment.

In the event you see your provider for a wellness visit and a problem is found, both a wellness code and diagnosis code can be submitted to your insurance company. It is important to note that insurance policies vary, and they may or may not pay for both types of service. Also, the order in which the codes are listed can influence payment. If a preventive code is used, *it must be placed first in order for that part of the examination to be covered.*

For Medicare Part B recipients, the *Initial Preventive Physical Exam (IPPE),* commonly referred to as the "Welcome to Medicare" visit, is a one-time covered benefit that must be used within the first twelve months of enrollment. During the visit your provider will:

- Record and evaluate your medical and family history, current health conditions, and prescriptions

- Check your blood pressure, vision, weight, and height to get a baseline for your care
- Make sure you are up-to-date with preventive screenings and services, such as cancer screenings and vaccines
- Order further tests, depending on your general health and medical history

Medicare Part B also covers an annual Wellness Visit. You are eligible for this benefit once each year, after you have had Part B for at least 12 months. The purpose of the Annual Wellness Visit is to develop or update your personalized prevention plan. *(See previously reviewed Wellness Exam.)*

Medical billing involves taking the coded information and making it into a bill, or *claim*. This process is used for all office visits, regardless of insurance status. For those patients with insurance, the healthcare system's Business Office sends the coded claim to the insurance company's Business Office. They then determine who much of it will be covered according to the patient's policy. This information is returned to the healthcare system's Business Office, who separates out how much of the bill is covered by insurance and how much the patient owes.

The healthcare system's biller takes into account the patient's *deductible, co-insurance, co-payment,* and *maximum out-of-pocket*. Much, if not all, of this information will be contained in the *Explanation of Benefits (EOB)*, a statement from your insurance company that summarizes the billed charges by all your providers and medical facilities, payments made by your insurance company, prescription payments, and the estimate of what is owed by you. A bill for the remaining amount is then sent to the patient. If the patient does not pay their bill, the healthcare system's biller has the authority to hire a collections agency.

If your claim is denied for payment, you will receive a letter from your insurance company stating so and why. Should this happen, begin by calling the Business Office of your *insurance company*. Tell them you received a letter denying the claim for the stated reason. Have the insurance company look up the code used and confirm why it was denied. It is possible for an insurance company to deny a claim based on the code used by the healthcare system. Likewise, if you are billed for a "Preventive Health" service (these will be discussed in Chapter 7), contact your insurance company's Business Office and confirm that the service provided does indeed fall under "Preventive Health" and is at no cost to you.

If the problem *can* be fixed by correcting the code, call the billing office of the *clinic that sent the bill*. Tell them you talked to the insurance company and relate what was said. (You can also have the insurance company contact the clinic, but it doesn't hurt to do your own follow-up.) Sometimes just a corrected code adjustment can make the difference between the insurance company covering the claim and you having to pay.

Any time you are attempting to resolve an insurance or medical conflict, always document who you talked to, when you talked to them, what their title is, and the method of correspondence (phone, email, letter, text). Include a summary of your conversation.

If your health insurance company refuses to pay a claim, you have the right to appeal their decision and have it reviewed by a third party. Should you decide to do this, contact your insurance company and ask how to initiate an *Appeals Process*. They will tell you what you need to know, what information to gather, and how to submit the request for review. The insurance company website may also contain this information.

If you do not have insurance, the bill will be sent directly to your mailing address. In the event you do not have the money to pay the bill, contact the Business Office to see what options are available to you, such as making monthly payments. Ask if there are resources available to help you pay your bill, or to apply for insurance or assistance. The clinic can refuse to see you again until it is paid.

Treatment of the Elderly

A special relationship should exist between the elderly patient and their provider.

The aged have reached the end stage of their lives. They are likely to have many health problems, take many medications, and have more than one provider. Most desire to stay as well as they can for as long as possible, and will do what is necessary to achieve this outcome. Many elderly individuals put their faith in their providers to give them the best possible care, because many times they have no one else to trust or turn to.

Still, the elderly are in a place where change complicates every aspect of living. It can be difficult for them to keep up. Having a provider who will listen to, and acknowledge, their concerns can be the key to their good health and well-being.

From a provider's perspective, treating an elderly patient can have its challenges. Because of their age, their body's ability to break down and absorb medications is altered. They are at an increased risk for side effects from the medications they take. There are changes, too, in an elderly patient's sleep, appetite and diet, activity level, hearing, and memory – all of which can affect their health. Yet many times, the provider will be unaware of these changes, as they may only see this patient every one to three months for a fifteen-minute visit.

Thus the relationship between the elderly patient and their provider requires a great deal of communication, observation, and listening by both parties involved. For it to be at its most effective, this may require the use of additional resources, such as trusted family members, Social Services/Care Management, home healthcare, and Hospice care. (*Social Services/Care Management* offer a variety of programs to individuals and families who need special assistance, such as with education, medical care, and housing. Medical services include patient education, medication management and adherence support, and coordination of care transition, such as from hospital to nursing home.)

Author's Note: If your provider wishes to do a multitude of testing, or testing that requires much preparation and will be hard for you to endure, make sure you, a family member, or a loved one understands the reasoning for it. Consider ahead of time, should the test have a bad report, if you will be agreeable or able to complete the treatment. And if so, what impact will it have on your quality of life.

Developing the Best Possible Relationship With a Provider

For all patients, having a mutual understanding between you and your provider is the best-case scenario. To accomplish this, both you and your provider must recognize that there may be some essential differences between how you regard your provider and how your provider perceives you.

Providers have had many years of training in order to provide quality healthcare to their patients. Every day they go to work and see a full schedule of patients who have health concerns. They are constantly thinking of what would benefit each individual patient. Patients, on the other hand, primarily seek healthcare because there is a problem - a problem they can't fix themselves. Or, they are trying to prevent a health problem from occurring, desiring to stay as healthy as possible. And sometimes they feel they are seeing a provider because they *have* to, not because they *want* to. For many patients, the goal is to get in quickly, solve the problem, and then get out. *Meeting in the middle, and together developing the best possible solution for maximum health, should be the goal in healthcare.*

Here are some practical tips that can help promote a positive relationship between you and your provider:

- *If you have trouble understanding what your provider just said, immediately ask them to explain it, or ask the medical assistant after the provider leaves.* Some patients feel intimidated by their provider, and are afraid to ask a question. If that is the case, consider ways that will increase communication, such as asking the medical assistant the question when you are placed in the room. They will document your concern, and the provider will expect the question - or even may bring the issue up once they read the assistant's note. Or write down your question on a piece of paper and hand it to the medical assistant for your provider to read before they come in. If you experience difficulty in understanding what is being said because of your provider's accent, let them know so they can speak slower, and more distinctly

- *If you find that you don't really like your provider and are thinking about changing, think about the reasons why first.* Consider if the problem is related to their bedside manner (how nice they are to you), the quality of their care (how well you feel they are taking care of your problem), or both. This may help you to decide what to do. If you decide to leave your provider, try to avoid doing so until you have secured a new provider. Once you leave a clinic practice, you may not be able to go back. Also, it may be more difficult to change providers from *within the same clinic practice.* However, if you desire to do so, speak with the receptionist about scheduling with the new provider. They will advise you of the clinic policy regarding this

- *Yes, your provider is a well-educated and trained medical professional, but you still need to understand that they may not be able to explain every single ache, pain, tingling, or unusual sensation you have.* Vague symptoms such as these can be a sign for a multitude of illnesses - or a sign of nothing at all. Be specific when describing your symptoms, and when asking any questions concerning them

- *If the provider asks you do so something, do it.* While you may not always understand the technical reasoning behind the request, your provider does. Again, don't be afraid to ask questions

- *If your health problem is a work-in-progress, such as control of your blood pressure or blood sugar, keep a record of your home readings and bring it to each office visit.* This helps your provider to see how you have doing in between visits, and helps them to decide a plan of care

- *Don't be unrealistic and expect the provider to remember all the medications you take, or what was talked about at your last appointment.* While you may only be seeing one provider, your provider sees many patients

- *Be cautious about believing statements made by healthcare providers that appear in the media.* This includes information given by medical professionals on talk shows, and research findings that you hear about through news anchors. While much of what they say may be true, some of what they say may not apply to you and your personal medical history. Before making healthcare decisions based on media hype, consult with your provider to determine if the information would be beneficial or dangerous to your health. Remember, you provider is more familiar with your health than anyone else

- *If your primary care provider manages the bulk of your healthcare, and yet now is referring you to a specialist, do not react defensively or angrily to this news.* They are not recommending this change in healthcare strategy because they don't like you or no longer want to see you. They are endorsing another professional with the expectation that you are going to receive more specialized care. They are looking out for you, and are trying to get you the very best care for your individual case. Keep in mind it is not uncommon to have more than one specialist

- *If you are unhappy with your specialist's care, secure another specialist before leaving the first.* Specialty providers can be more difficult to get into. They tend to practice in groups, and there are only so many groups available

And here's a bit more on specialists...

If You Need to See a Specialist

Many specialists will only manage illnesses related to their specialty. For example, your Cardiologist (heart specialist) may not remove the stitches you received while in the Urgent Care, or your Podiatrist (foot specialist) may not treat your sinus infection.

Each specialist has their own billing system as well. So if the provider orders a chest x-ray, you will receive two bills - one from the facility where the chest x-ray was done, and the other from the Radiologist who read the x-ray. Likewise, if you have a skin cancer removed, the Dermatologist will send a bill for the procedure, and the Pathologist who looked at the skin sample under the microscope will send another.

If the Urgent Care or Emergency Room refers you to Specialist A but you want to see Specialist B, you can do so assuming Specialist B agrees to see you. If you have insurance, check to see if Specialist B is covered in your plan. Remember, you are responsible for scheduling most referral appointments to a specialist.

If your provider refers you to Specialist A when Specialist B is closer and more convenient, don't hesitate to discuss this with your provider. If your provider has no specific reason for referring you to Specialist A, they may just as well refer you to Specialist B. But if your provider feels strongly about you seeing Specialist A, try to make every accommodation to do so.

You have the option to obtain a *"second opinion"* about your healthcare advice should you feel it necessary. Some providers will be supportive of this decision, and some insurance plans will cover the cost. If you are unsure, call your insurance plan's Patient Services representative prior to making any appointment to ask if they cover the cost of seeking out a second opinion.

If a specialist performs a medical procedure on you - putting a feeding tube into your stomach, putting a cast on your leg, or placing a port under your skin for chemotherapy – the general rule is to follow-up with that specialist. Whoever puts it in/on will most likely want to take it out/off. If the procedure is done in the Emergency Room, such as stitches, you will be instructed on where and when to follow-up when you are discharged.

Throughout the territory of healthcare, your primary care provider (PCP) is at the center of your health. Ultimately, they are responsible for coordinating all your healthcare needs, whether it is in their office or referring you to a specialist. If your PCP refers you to a specialist, the specialist should send your PCP a report stating the diagnosis and plan of care after seeing you, so your PCP will know what is going on with you. If your insurance does not require you to have a PCP and/or you chose not to have one, let me remind you of the benefits of having one. Your primary care provider:

- Identifies and treats common medical conditions
- Provides preventive care (e.g., screenings and check-ups) and promotes healthy lifestyle choices
- Assesses the urgency of your medical problems and directs you to the best place for that care
- Makes referrals to medical specialists when necessary

If you would like to see a certain specialist, first talk to your PCP about it. While some insurance companies do not require you to have a referral to see a specialist, many do. Those companies that require a referral want you and your PCP to make the decision together. For example, let's say you have a skin problem and are concerned about a skin cancer, but have never established with an in-network Dermatologist (skin specialist). In this scenario, you schedule to see your PCP first. If they feel you need to be seen by a specialist, they will refer you to a Dermatologist. Once you have established with the Dermatologist, you have the option to be seen again by them for future skin concerns, without going through your PCP.

Your Specialist will document their findings and treatments in your electronic health record (EHR), which your PCP can review. If no EHR is available, it is likely some type of correspondence will be sent from the specialist to the referring provider. Moreover, some specialists may not agree to see you without a referral from your PCP. It is important for them to know that you have first been evaluated by your PCP and are in need of specialty care.

While certain insurance companies may not pay for your specialist office visit without a referral, there are also insurance companies that need to approve the PCP's referral – before you can be seen by the specialist!

However, there are exceptions to this rule and a referral may not be necessary for the following specialty areas:

- Obstetrician/Gynecologist (OB/GYN): Women's healthcare needs, such as a Pap test or pregnancy. Going to an OB/GYN who is covered by your insurance usually does not require a referral
- Behavioral (mental) health issues: Review your insurance plan to see if a referral is necessary
- Emergency Room visits: The Emergency Room provider can refer you to a specialist without you being seen by your PCP first

CHAPTER 5

Medications
(More is not always better)

One of the areas of healthcare that is the most confusing to consumers is medication (e.g., drugs, pills, or medicine). A very long book could be written just on this subject alone! In this book, however, I will focus on basic information about medication as it applies to the general patient.

The goals of medication are to:

- Prevent disease,
- Cure illness, and
- Promote health.

The FDA's Role

Because the U.S. Food and Drug Administration (FDA) plays such a crucial role when it comes to medications, let's first take a moment to see exactly what this agency does.

The origins of the U.S. Food and Drug Administration as a federal consumer protection agency began with the passage of the 1906 Pure Food and Drugs Act. This law was the end product of about 100 bills that aimed to rein in long-standing, serious abuses in the consumer product marketplace. The FDA is an agency within the U.S. Department of Health and Human Services. It consists of the Office of the Commissioner and four cabinets that oversee the core functions of the agency: Medical Products and Tobacco, Foods and Veterinary Medicine, Global Regulatory Operations and Policy, and Operations. The FDA is responsible for:

- Protecting the public health by assuring that foods (except for meat from livestock, poultry and some egg products which are regulated by the U.S. Department of Agriculture) are safe, wholesome, sanitary, and properly labeled
- Ensuring that medications, vaccines, and other biological products and medical devices intended for human use are safe and effective
- Protecting the public from electronic product radiation
- Assuring cosmetics and dietary supplements are safe and properly labeled
- Regulating tobacco products
- Advancing the public health by helping to speed product innovations

Understanding Different Medication Types

Medications you can buy without needing a provider's authorization (or prescription) are commonly referred to as *over-the-counter (OTC)* medications. Some common types of OTC medication include aspirin, *Claritin^R*, *Pepto-Bismol^R*, and *Lotrimin^R* Antifungal cream. It is very important to read the OTC drug's label. It tells you what the medication is supposed to do, who should and shouldn't take it, and how to use it. Per FDA guidelines, the following information must appear in the following order:

- *Active ingredient:* The product's active ingredients, including the amount in each dosage unit
- *Purpose:* Product action or category
- *Uses:* Symptoms or diseases the product will treat or prevent
- *Warnings:* When the product should not be used under any circumstances, and when it is appropriate to consult with a doctor or pharmacist. This section also describes side effects that can occur and substances or activities to avoid
- *Directions:* Specific age categories, how much to take, how to take, how often, and for how long
- *Inactive ingredients:* Important information to help consumers avoid ingredients that may cause an allergic reaction *(this will be discussed shortly)*
- *Other:* Expiration date, lot or batch code, manufacturer, how much of the product is in each package, and what to do if an overdose occurs

However, many medications require a prescription, which is given to you by your provider or forwarded by your provider to your pharmacy of choice.

Whether a medication is available over-the-counter or through a prescription, it has a history behind its availability. New medications can be developed for a specific disease, or they may be discovered by accident. It can take eleven to fourteen years for an *Investigational New Drug* to be developed in the lab and tested on human beings before being approved for marketing by the FDA. And, according to the Tufts Center for the Study of Drug Development (2014), it costs nearly $2.6 billion to develop a new drug that gains marketing approval. A *New Drug Application* includes all the animal and human data (*clinical trials*), analysis of this data, information on how the drug works in the body, and how it is manufactured.

When a drug is first discovered, it is given a chemical name which describes its atomic or molecular formula. After the drug has been approved by the FDA, it is assigned a *generic (official)* name by the U.S. Adopted Names Council. Every medication has a generic name. The name reflects the *class* that the drug is in. The *class*, or *category*, describes how the medication works. Medications that work in a similar manner are placed in the same class.

When a brand new medication is ready to be sold to the public, it is given a *brand-name (proprietary; trademark; trade)*. This is a name given by the drug company that has exclusive rights to selling it. They also receive a patent on the product which protects their rights to it. Because the drug company owns the medication, they can name it what they like, and be the only company that sells it. The original brand type is called the *index pill*.

Once the patent expires on a brand-named drug (most drug patents are protected for twenty years), the drug is allowed to be manufactured and sold as generic. This means the original drug company can no longer be the only company that makes this particular medication. Multiple companies can manufacture the medication if they so choose. These companies can sell the drug by its generic name, or even give it a new *brand-name*. Medications are then sorted into categories according to *indication*, or diagnosis.

For example:

Class: Contraception
Brand | *Index* name: *Ortho-Tri-Cyclen*[R]
Molecular Formula: $C_{43}H_{55}NO_5$
Generic | Brand: Norgestimate/ethinyl estradiol; *Tri-Estarylla*[R]; *TriSprintec*[R]; *TriNessa*[R]
Indication (Diagnosis): Family Planning

While it is common to hear concerns about how well generic medications work compared to the brand-name product, the FDA offers research-based reassurance about any generic versions that are made available:

1. Generic drugs must meet rigorous standards with respect to identity, strength, quality, purity, and potency.
2. Generic drugs are required to have the same active (main) ingredient(s), strength, dosage form, and route of administration (e.g., pill, liquid, inhaled, shot, patch, cream/ointment) as the brand-name, or original, drug.
3. The generic drug manufacturer must prove its drug is the same as the brand-name drug.
4. All generic manufacturing, packaging, and testing sites must pass the same quality standards as those of brand-name drugs.
5. The generic products must meet the same exacting specifications as any brand- name product. Many generic drugs are made in the same manufacturing plants as brand-name drug products.

A Cautionary Word on Dietary Supplements

According to the FDA, "a dietary supplement is a product intended for ingestion that contains a 'dietary ingredient' intended to add further nutritional value to supplement the diet." This includes vitamins, minerals, herbs or other botanicals, amino acids, substances to increase total dietary intake, a concentrate, metabolite, constituent, or extract, or any combination thereof.

Herbal medication - a type of dietary supplement - is a plant (or part of a plant) used for its scent, flavor, and/or healing properties. Herbal supplements come in many forms: tablets, capsules, powders, teas, extracts, and fresh or dried plants. Many people choose to use *herbal supplements* to maintain or improve their health. Many of these consumers believe that products labeled *"natural"* – as herbal supplements usually are – are always safe and good for them, but, that is not necessarily true. Herbal medicines do *not* go through the FDA's rigorous testing that standard medications do, because they are considered a food, and fall under the "dietary supplement" category. Some herbs can cause serious harm, while other herbs can interact with prescription or over-the-counter medications.

Before a company markets a dietary supplement, they are responsible for ensuring that the product(s) it manufactures and/or distributes is safe, and claims made about the product are not false or misleading. Nutritional information must be included on the label. The active ingredient must also be stated. Unlike drugs, dietary supplements are not intended to treat, diagnose, prevent, or cure diseases.

It is very important for your provider to know *every* medication you are taking, whether or not it is prescription. This includes herbal medications, vitamins, body-building supplements, and over-the-counter-medications. So if you are thinking about using a dietary supplement, first review doing so with your provider. Add them to your medication list and report them to all your healthcare providers. Realize that if you are being seen by any providers and/or specialist outside of the provider's health system, the EHR (electronic health record) may not have a record of them.

Author's Note: Some providers prefer that you bring all your medications with you to each of your office visits so that they can review the medication, dose, and refill status.

What's Coupled with Your Medication

It is important to realize that when you take a medication, it is not just a drug you are taking in. *Additives*, also known as *inactive ingredients*, are mixed with the drug to make it easier to swallow, or to help it to break up in the stomach or intestines, for example. Inactive ingredients are usually harmless and do not affect the body. (There may be a few people, however, that can be allergic to a specific additive.) The type and amount of additives, and the degree of pill density, affect how quickly the swallowed tablet breaks down and is absorbed. Here are some examples of how additives are used:

- If a pill is irritating to the stomach, it can be coated with an additive so it doesn't break down until it reaches the small intestine. This is called *enteric-coated*
- Some pills are specially made with the help of additives to release their active ingredients slowly over time. These pills are called *controlled-release, sustained-release,* or *extended-release*
- Additives can provide bulk so that a tablet is large enough to handle
- Additives keep a tablet from crumbling between the time it is made and the time it is used by the patient
- Additives can give the medication a pleasant taste and color

Because generic medications may use different inactive ingredients, absorption of the drug may vary between the generic and the brand-name version. According to FDA research, the average difference of absorption into the body between the generic and the brand-name is 3.5 percent.

Essential Information When You Start Taking a Medication

When any medication is taken, whether it is OTC (over-the-counter) or by prescription, it is important that you be aware of all the following information. In fact, you should keep this information easily available to you as long as you take your medication. (*Author's Note:* Much of this medication information can be found on the package labeling, in the papers attached to the prescription bag, or by talking with your provider or your pharmacist):

- *Why:* Why are you taking this medication? If you are taking multiple medications, or just only one, consider asking your provider to include your diagnosis on your prescription. This will then be added to your prescription label, helping you to remember why you are taking each medication

- *Name:* What name is on the label? Is it the generic name, the brand name, or are both names on the label?

- *Dose:* What dose should you be taking? Dosages are given usually in the following measurements: mg (milligram); g (gram); milliliter (mL); microgram (mcg); and milliequivalent (mEq). This information can be found on the medication label.

  (*Author's Note:* The unit of measurement [mg, gram, mL, mcg, mEq] for one type of medication is not comparable to a unit of measure for a different type of medication. For example, Medication A, that is a 10 mg dose, is not comparable to Medication B, in a 1000 mg dose. Medication B is not considered "stronger" just because it has more milligrams (mg). It is what the specific drug is made of, and how the body uses it, that determines the strength

- *Frequency:* How often are you to take the medication? For example, it may be that you should take it three times a day, or that you should be taking it *just as needed* (also known as PRN: pro re nata = as the circumstance arises)

- *Route of administration*: Should you take it by mouth; apply it to the skin; put in the rectum, vagina, or ears/eyes/nose; inhale; or inject it one of three ways (subcutaneous [SQ] – into the fat layer, intradermal – just under the skin, or intramuscular [IM] - into the muscle)
- *Duration*: Are you to take the drug on a *short term* basis, e.g., for only one day or for a few days, such as with an antibiotic – or for the *long term*, e.g., take it every day, for the rest of your life, to treat a long-term condition, such as high blood pressure or diabetes
- *Environment*: What type of environment is best for the medicine? For example, as the drug might be sensitive to heat or cold, you might need to keep the medication at room temperature or in the refrigerator. Or, you might need to protect it from sunlight
- *Prescriber*: What is the name of the provider or specialist who prescribes the medication?
- *When*: When are you to take it? Should you be taking it first thing in the morning, or at bedtime? And, how important is it for you to take at the same time each day?
- *How*: How are you to take it? For example, should you be taking it on an empty stomach, or with food?
- *Expiration Date*: When does the medication expire? This should be printed on the medication prescription label
- *Allergies*: Are you allergic to this medication? If so, what was the reaction, and when did it occur?

Medication and Your Pharmacy

Once you and your provider have discussed starting a new medication or refilling another, you will need to go about filling your prescription. First let's review where you will get your medication from:

1. Mail-order Pharmacy (for those with insurance)
   - Affiliated with your insurance company
   - Online ordering (billed to your credit card or Health Savings Account [HSA] credit card. HSA is part of a higher-deductible type of insurance that issues a credit/debit card for payment)

- Three month (ninety-day) refills
- Most cost-effective for long-term medications
- Automatic refills: The company will send an email that the medication has been filled, and/or when the medication is sent
- If you do not choose the option of automatic refills, the company may send you a reminder email, asking if you want to refill your prescription
- You may have the option to instruct the mail-order pharmacy to contact your provider for refills, if none are available
- Medicare requires that mail-order services (when filling or refilling medications for Medicare patients) call and confirm that you want the desired medication before it is shipped

2. Neighborhood Pharmacy (with or without insurance)
   - Short to long-term medications – one dose to years of use
   - Offers monthly refills or three month (ninety-day) refills on many long-term medications
   - When you sign up for automatic refills, the pharmacy will contact you when your medication is ready for pick-up, contact the provider if refills are needed, and continue to refill the medication until you request they stop
   - Phone apps may be available for medication management

3. Provider-dispensed medication
   - The rules and regulations vary from state to state, so talk to your provider to see what may be available to you

Secondly, getting the prescription to the desired pharmacy can be done several ways:

1. *Your provider or their assistant can send the prescription through the computer from your EHR (electronic health record).* This can go to the requested neighborhood pharmacy or directly to the mail-order pharmacy.
2. *Your provider or their assistant can call in the prescription by telephone.* When the call is made to a neighborhood pharmacy, the prescription message is typically left on the pharmacy's answering machine. The provider or the assistant also has the option to speak directly with a pharmacist, if the medication needs to be filled right away or if there are questions or comments. If

the call is made to the mail-order company, many times the provider or their assistant will speak directly to the pharmacist.

3. *They can receive the prescription by fax.* The provider or the assistant can send a signed order by fax to the pharmacy, or the pharmacy can request a medication refill by sending a fax to your clinic, which the provider signs and sends back.

4. *You may receive hand-written or computer-printed prescriptions made available by some clinic practices.* These either may be handed directly to you (for example, if you are at an appointment, or if you call to alert the staff that you need a new prescription and ask when you can stop by to pick it up), or mailed to you at your address on record.

For those with insurance, keep in mind that the medical and pharmacy coverage may be provided by two different companies, meaning there may be two different cards, two sets of information, and two different websites for you to access. Although the companies work together for you, they provide you with different services.

If you are new to the mail-order service, you must first register at the pharmacy website, which includes giving them your credit card or HSA account number for payment. Your provider may then call in or fax all prescriptions once they have the contact information, or you may be requested to mail in the actual prescription(s).

If you have insurance and wish to pick up your medication at your *neighborhood pharmacy*, be sure and check with the insurance (or pharmacy) company about which pharmacies are covered under you plan. Covered pharmacies can be found at the insurance (or pharmacy) company website under *Pharmacy* or *Prescription Benefits* (or under some other similar language.) However, you may not be able to obtain this information until you have registered with the company website (insurance or pharmacy). You also can call your insurance company's Customer Service for this information.

(For those without insurance, finding a pharmacy and paying for medication will be discussed later in this chapter.)

The paperwork and label attached to your prescription includes important information, such as when to take the medication in regard to meals, or side effects to watch for (more about this later in the chapter). Review this before you leave the store to make sure you understand the instructions, and if not, ask. Or, if you read the paperwork and find it contains information that may make you not want to take the medication, discuss these concerns with your pharmacist or provider.

The information on your prescription label will include:

- The name of the medication (brand and/or generic)
- The number of units in the prescription (the number of pills, for example)
- Directions for its use (how much and how often)
- The date dispensed
- The medication's expiration date
- The number of refills available and the refill expiration date (The last day the medication can be refilled)
- The pharmacy phone number
- The prescription number

When the medication is in pill form, the label will be attached to the bottle the pills come in. When the medication is in another form, such as a suppository, eye drops, or skin cream, the label may be attached to the medication container. It is important to keep your medication in the container it comes in, so that you have the label information available to you.

Understanding Prescription Labels and the Refill Process

Once you are in the possession of your medication, it is very important you keep track of how much you receive, how much you have used, and how many refills you have left. The last thing you and your provider want is for you to run out of medication. In some cases, abruptly stopping medication can worsen or be dangerous to your health.

You can help keep track of the amount of medication available to you by looking at the label, which will state the number of medication refills available to you. Each time the medication is refilled, the pharmacy updates how many refills remain available to you on the most current label.

If you have refills available and choose to use the option for automatic refills, your neighborhood pharmacy will call when your medication is ready for pick-up, or your mail-order pharmacy will confirm with you online that you want to refill a specific medication and/or notify you when the medication has been shipped.

Your insurance company decides how soon you can refill a long-term prescription at your neighborhood pharmacy. Some companies allow the pharmacy to dispense a medication refill seven days before it is needed, while others limit the time your pharmacy can dispense your medication to only twenty-four hours ahead of time. There are also some insurance companies that require the patient to refill their medication at a neighborhood pharmacy every twenty-one to twenty-eight days. By doing this, the insurance company is encouraging the patient to use the mail-order option, which is more cost-effective to the company. (Know that the refill protocol is stricter with narcotic medications, which will be discussed later in this chapter.) In addition, when filling a prescription at your neighborhood pharmacy, some insurance companies will only allow the pharmacist to dispense one month at a time, while other companies will allow dispensing three months at a time.

When filling your long-term prescription medication at your neighborhood pharmacy for the first time, ask the pharmacy technician to look and see how soon you can refill the medication and if you have the option of receiving three months of medication at a time. Having this information will help you to plan your next refill before running out of medication. If you do not choose to use an automatic refill option, you should contact your neighborhood pharmacy when you have one week of monthly medication left or one to two weeks of medication left for three month refills.

For mail-order medication refills (three months of medication), contact your on-line pharmacy when you have two to four weeks of medication left. They should be able to advise you on how soon you can refill your medication. Some mail-order websites will show how many refills you have left and when you can refill the prescription. Know that some mail-order pharmacies will not leave medication of any type unattended at the front door. They require someone to accept the package. This could be your next-door neighbor or a scheduled pick-up at the delivery company's business.

When you have no refills left, the label may read "0 refills" or "no refills left". *The best time to obtain refills for your medication from your provider is when you have received the last refill.* Keep in mind that your provider may need to see you before your medication can be refilled - which may require some time, so allow time for both making the appointment and being seen. (It will be all too easy to forget to do this as the days pass.) If you have signed up for automatic refills, your pharmacy (neighborhood or mail-order) may inform you when there are no more refills available. They may offer to contact your provider for refills, or encourage you to do so. Also, realize it also may take time for a mail-order pharmacy to process the refill order, so build that into your time frame as well.

If you find you will run out of medication before receiving the mail-order pharmacy medication, consider requesting your provider call into your neighborhood pharmacy for one month's worth of medication, to fill in the gap so you do not run out completely. If your insurance company will not pay for a double refill request (the same prescription filled both at the online pharmacy *and* the neighborhood pharmacy), ask the neighborhood pharmacy how much it will cost you out-of-pocket for the specific number of pills you need, until your mail-order pharmacy refill arrives. Purchase what you are able, so as not to run out medication.

Here are the ways to obtain a medication refill:

1. Contact the neighborhood pharmacy where the prescription was originally filled, and have them request a refill order from your provider, *OR*
2. Go to your mail-order website and have them request a refill order from your provider, *OR*
3. Call your provider's office to have them call refills to your neighborhood pharmacy or mail-order service.

When you are calling about your need for a refill, listen for the "medication refill" option of the phone message. Whether you leave a medication refill-request message, talk to your provider's office, or speak with the mail-order or neighborhood pharmacy representative, have the following information on hand:

- Your name
- Date of birth
- Call back number
- Name and dose of medication
- The prescription number (if calling the pharmacy)
- Where the prescription is to be filled (e.g., the name and phone number of your local pharmacy or the mail-order company)

Having this information on hand will quicken the process, should you be asked for it. It may help if you write this information on a separate piece of paper for easy reference.

From a provider's perspective, it is very frustrating when a patient calls the clinic saying they ran out of their medication yesterday and need a refill prescription today. Keeping track of how many pills and refills you have left, and calling in for a refill with plenty of time for the provider to sign off on it and get it to you or your pharmacy, will keep both you and your provider happy.

It is common practice for providers to require twenty-four business-day hours for medication refills. That means refill requests called to the provider at the end of their clinic day will most likely be taken care of the following work day. Know too that if you call late Friday afternoon for a refill and the clinic is closed on weekends, you may not be able to get it filled until Monday. Plan ahead for long holiday weekends, when your provider's office may be closed and unavailable for medication refill requests.

As previously mentioned, providers have an ethical and legal obligation to their patients. So if a patient on medication chooses not to keep their follow-up appointments, the provider cannot know how well the patient is doing or if medication changes are needed. And certain diagnoses and medications require more frequent follow-ups. So schedule and keep your follow-up appointments. This strengthens the patient-provider relationship and guarantees quality medication management. In so doing, you will not run the risk of your provider refusing to refill your medication because you have not been seen at the requested intervals.

Realize, too, it is not unusual to go pick up a refill at your neighborhood pharmacy that your provider has called in to, only to discover that the order is not yet ready. Getting upset with the pharmacy tech because your prescription isn't ready doesn't help matters. Remain patient. It takes time to process all the prescriptions, and your pharmacy handles many prescription requests and many customers. Consider calling ahead of time, to see if your prescription is ready for pick-up. Or, if applicable, utilize the automatic refill option. You will be notified when your prescription is ready for pick-up.

Price Matters

Of all the steps necessary to obtain your prescription medication, paying for it can be the most challenging. Brand-name medications that are new to the market can be quite costly. Older medications, that have been on the market for several years and are being manufactured by many companies (generic), can cost very little. For patients who are taking several medications, the burden is even greater.

For those with insurance, medication coverage differs among companies. Most have a list of preferred medications that are less expensive for their members. (Many generic medications fall under this umbrella). An insurance company's medication list is often tiered, from least expensive, to very expensive, to not covered at all - meaning you will have to pay for all of it. So before you fill a new prescription through your insurance, research it to see if it is covered under your plan, and at what level. This can be done by searching on the pharmacy (or insurance) website for the *Formulary*, which is a list of covered medications. (The cost of the medication may also be listed there.) Some websites also offer the option of comparing similar medications and their prices or showing a less expensive option for a medication that is not covered or is very expensive. There may be an option to "Price Medication", where you will need to enter the name, dose, and frequency. Or, you can have your neighborhood pharmacy run the prescription through your insurance company.

If your provider desires to begin a medication that is not covered by your insurance company and you are unable to afford it, ask your provider about initiating a *"Prior Authorization"* request with the insurance (or pharmacy) company to help get the medication paid for. It is your provider's responsibility to complete the application. This may take some time but the result may be worth it.

There may be a time when your provider wishes to begin a new (and usually more expensive) medication after other medications have failed. Be open-minded should your provider offer you medication samples. *Medication samples* are new, brand-name medications given to health clinics by the drug companies. This is a great (and inexpensive) way to determine if a medication will improve your health without having to pay for one that may not help. Drug companies provide such samples hoping that if you respond positively to the new medication, you will be more inclined to continue taking it (and then paying for it). A *Prior Authorization* request can also be started in a case like this.

For those who have no or inadequate insurance coverage, finding affordable medications can certainly complicate healthcare. If your provider wants to start you on a medication and you can't afford it, talk to them about other options. This would include:

1. *Similar generic medications*: Many pharmacies offer a variety of very inexpensive generic medications. Call around to the different pharmacies and compare prices. There are also a handful of free medications available at certain pharmacies.
2. *Medication samples for short-term use.*
3. *Patient Assistant Programs*: You may be able to get free or low-cost brand-name drugs directly from the company that makes them. Enrollment can be started online but paperwork will still need to be filled out and signed by you and your provider. Additional information on your financial status may also be required. To see if you are eligible, go to the website of the drug company

that makes the requested brand-name drug. (The name of the company can be found on the prescription bottle. Or search for it on the Internet after you plug in the drug name.) Then search for *"Patient Assistance Program"* at the pharmaceutical company website.

4. *Prescription drug discount programs*: You may be able to get reduced prices on your medications through a free discount program. Pharmacies, as well as independent companies, provide discounts on many generic and brand-name medications. Some require enrollment, some do not. Talk with your provider or pharmacist for more information.

5. *Safety net providers*: Pharmacies in certain government-funded hospitals, community clinics, and health centers may provide medication at a reduced price or through a system based on income (sliding scale).

Tips on Remembering to Take Your Medication

When it comes time to take your newly refilled generic medication, you may notice that the pills or liquid looks differently from the previous order. There may be a simple explanation for this. When pharmacies buy generic medications in bulk, they will look for the least expensive price, and/or may purchase from several different manufacturers. Each manufacturer may offer a different color or shape (due to in-active ingredients), although *the medication will contain the same active ingredient*. Still, it is always wise to contact your pharmacy if your pills look differently. It does no harm to make sure that you have the correct medication.

Taking the medication as prescribed can sometimes be a challenge, especially if taken several times a day. Here are some ideas to help you remember:

1. *Purchase a pill box*, which come in quite a variety. For example, there are boxes ranging from weekly to monthly and from once-a day to four times a-day medication. The day of the week is often printed on the top of each compartment. Using a pill box every day will help you to *see* if you took your pills or not.

2. *Leave reminder notes* in as many places it takes to help you to remember.

3. *Set an alarm* in your phone, download a medication reminder app, or set a clock alarm or timer.

4. *Combine your pill-taking with a daily task*, such as brushing teeth or drinking your morning coffee. Set the medication bottle near to the daily task.

5. *Leave the medications in visible sight*.

6. *Ask a loved one to help you remember.*
7. *If the medication needs to be taken with a meal, set the bottle on the table near where you eat.*
8. *Write with marker on the cap of the bottle to remind you how often the pill needs to be taken per day, such as "AM" or "PM".*
9. *Place a few pills in a safe place you frequent, such as in your office, car, or purse.* If you happen to forget to take your medicine in the morning, you can easily take your medication later in the day if you have it near to you.

Even with all the good intentions, there will be times when you miss a dose. Now what? This is a difficult question. There are too many factors that influence the answer. For example:

- Medications are metabolized in different parts of the body at different rates. Some stay in the body a long time, while others are absorbed and utilized very quickly
- The age of the patient, their weight, the type of illness, the number of medications they take, and how the medication is taken (e.g., by mouth, inhaled, injected, or placed on the skin) can affect how quickly a medication is metabolized
- Some medications must be exactly dosed to keep blood levels at a certain number
- Some medications must be taken at precisely the same time every day for maximum effectiveness

So the best answer to the question? When your medication is prescribed during the office visit or when you realize you've missed a dose, ask your provider or pharmacist what you should do. Write down the answer to this question on your medication list to prevent future confusion.

Dos and Don'ts about Taking Half a Pill

In certain instances, it may be recommended that you take *only half a pill*. This could occur when a lower dose is needed, or to reduce costs. Pill splitting is not for all pills and all people, however. So talk to your provider or pharmacist to see if this is an option for you before embarking on this plan of care.

If you are considering taking half a pill or have been instructed to do so, here is some helpful information:

- If your pill has an indented line down the middle (this is called "*scored*"), the pill can be safely broken in half. Pills that are made to be split have been formulated to have equal amounts of medication on each side. Scored tablets can be broken in two relatively easily using your fingers. However, there are some pills that can safely be split that are not scored
- Do NOT try to cut pills that are not meant to be split. This includes most controlled-release, sustained-release, and long acting medications. Breaking pills that are not meant to be split may mean one side may not contain the dose of medication that you need – or may contain too much. Long-acting medications are formulated for slow release into the body. Breaking the tablet open will allow the medication to be released into your body too quickly. Some long-acting medications, such as pain pills, can be lethal if broken in half and swallowed
- Do not try to break pills into one thirds or one fourths unless recommended to do so by your provider
- Do not split the entire supply of tablets at one time and then store them for later use. Factors, such as heat and humidity, can affect the split pill, causing it to be less effective or too strong
- A tablet splitter (available through your local pharmacy) may help you to split your pill cleanly, although no one size of splitter fits all pills
- If you are paying out-of-pocket for your prescription pills and the pills are scored, speak with your pharmacist or provider about changing the prescription pill dose, so that only one-half pill is needed. For example, let's say your prescription is for a 25mg tablet to be taken daily. The pharmacy has 25mg and 50mg tablets available, both of which of scored. If your provider writes the prescription for a 25mg tablet to be taken daily, you are paying for 30 tablets (1 month of medication). If your provider writes the prescription for a 50mg tablet with instructions to take one-half tablet daily, you will only need to buy 15 tablets per month, which will save you money. Using this example, for long-term medications, you would only need to purchase forty-five tablets for three months of medication. (For those purchasing their prescriptions through the insurance company, speak with your representative to see if this would be cost-saving for you)

- Discuss your pill-splitting options with your pharmacist or provider

Essential Information If You Stop Taking a Medication

If you are prescribed a medication and do not fill the prescription or choose to stop taking it, it is important you notify the provider who wrote the prescription. Inform them as to why you aren't taking it, as there may be an alternative your provider can recommend. For example, if the medicine is not affordable for you, the provider may be able to prescribe another medication that still treats your condition but is less expensive. If there are side effects that you can't tolerate, your provider needs to know, and they may be able to suggest another medication without the same side effects. If you stop taking the medication just because you don't want to take any more pills, the provider needs to know so they can make a change to your agreed-upon plan-of-care. Remember, there is a reason the provider has prescribed you a specific medication, and *in writing the prescription is only trying to improve your health*. After having prescribed the medication, the provider assumes you are taking it *unless you tell them otherwise*.

If it is your provider who decides that you should stop taking a medication, you may be at a loss with what to do with any remaining pills. The Federal Drug Administration (FDA) and the White House Office of National Drug Control Policy offers the following recommendations when disposing of medication: www.fda.gov/ForConsumers/ConsumerUpdates/ucm101653.htm.

Follow any specific disposal instructions on the prescription drug labeling or patient information that accompanies the medication. Do not flush medications down the sink or toilet unless this information specifically instructs you to do so.

1. Take advantage of community drug take-back programs that allow the public to bring unused drugs to a central location for proper disposal. Call or go to the website of your city or county government's household trash and recycling service (see blue pages in phone book) to see if a take-back program is available in your community.
2. If no disposal instructions are given on the prescription drug labeling and no take-back program is available in your area, throw the medications in the household trash following these steps:
   - Remove them from their original containers and mix them with an undesirable substance, such as used coffee grounds or cat litter. This makes

the medication less appealing to children and pets, and unrecognizable to people who may intentionally go through the trash seeking drugs

- Place the mixture in a sealable bag, an empty can, a jar with a lid, or another container to prevent the medication from leaking or breaking out of a garbage bag
- Before throwing out a medication container, scratch out all identifying information on the prescription label to make it unreadable, or completely remove the label and destroy it. This will help protect your identity and the privacy of your personal health information
- Do not give your medication to friends. Providers prescribe medications based on your specific symptoms and medical history. A medication that works for you could be dangerous for someone else
- When in doubt about proper disposal, talk to your pharmacist

Many households contain *narcotic prescriptions*. These medications are called "*controlled substances*" due to their potential for dependency (addiction) and abuse. Because narcotics are highly sought after by many kinds of people, there are some key things you should know concerning them:

- Providers are very cautious when writing narcotics, so you must take the narcotic medication as prescribed and refill it *no sooner than when your provider and pharmacist recommend*
- If you lose your narcotics or they are stolen, it may be difficult for you to get a refill
- If you are unable to personally pick up your prescription at the pharmacy, you may be given the option to name a person to pick them up for you. Should you choose to do this, select your person very carefully
- Whenever picking up a narcotic prescription, identification must be presented
- Count the pills when first filled, and periodically, to make sure that no one is "helping themselves" to your prescription medication
- Don't leave a narcotic pill bottle sitting out for people to see. If there will be strangers in your house - such as your house is for sale or repair people are coming - hide the pills or take them with you
- Don't advertise you are taking narcotics to others

- If you feel you are at risk of the medication being stolen, hide the bottle or keep it in a safe
- Don't keep the medication in a purse or car
- Prescription drugs, such as powerful narcotic pain relievers and other controlled substances, carry instructions for flushing down the toilet. Doing so reduces the danger of unintentional use and illegal abuse, for both pills and patches

When you pick up a prescription at your local pharmacy, the staff will often ask if there are any questions about the medication, regardless of your insurance status. *Make the most out of your pharmacy by taking advantage of the pharmacist's medical knowledge.* The pharmacist will be able to answer almost any or all questions - and will do so regardless of how embarrassing the questions may seem to you. Taking medication can be a serious matter, and having as much information as possible will ease your mind and promote well-being. So ask the question, if you have one. A sampling of store-front pharmacy services includes:

- If you have insurance and a new prescription, the pharmacy can run the new prescription through your insurance company and tell you how much it will cost
- Making automatic refills available on many long-term medications
- You may request the prescription bottle with or without child-resistant caps
- Your pills may come in a *blister pack*, where each pill is individually sealed in a month's sheet of pills. If you find it difficult to get the pills out, you can ask the pharmacy to place them in a bottle for you instead
- In the event your provider needs to be contacted for a refill, the pharmacy can call your provider for you. In this scenario, please allow the pharmacy twenty-four hours to get the medicine refilled for you
- If you will be traveling, plan ahead so you don't run out of your medication. For example, you can work with your pharmacy to see if you can get an early medication refill, or if you can get your prescription transferred to the local pharmacy branch where you will be staying. If your insurance company will not pay for an early refill to cover your travels, ask the pharmacy how much it will cost out-of-pocket for the specific number of pills you need, so you don't run out of medication

- Provides travel-size bottles for prescription and over-the-counter liquid medications
- Reviews potential drug interactions when two or more medications are taken. If the pharmacist becomes concerned about the combination of medications or a potential negative side effect, they can contact your provider with their concerns
- Offers vaccines, such as a tetanus, flu, or pneumonia shot
- Sells (or may rent) Durable Medical Equipment (DME). This would include walkers, crutches, shower stools, and nebulizers for breathing treatments
- May provide a walk-in Urgent Care
- Information and instruction on measuring tools for powder and liquid medications
- Will assist you in transferring your prescriptions to another pharmacy, if needed

There are some pharmacies that specialize in *compounding* medications. This means that a licensed pharmacist is able to combine, mix, or alter ingredients of a drug or drugs to create a medication tailored to the specific needs of a patient. Compounded medications are not FDA-approved, which means that the FDA does not verify the safety or effectiveness of compounded drugs. Yet, there are times when the healthcare needs of a patient can't be met by an FDA-approved medication. For example, if a patient has an allergy to a medication and needs it to be made without a certain dye (inactive ingredient), the pharmacist can compound a medication that the patient is not allergic to. Or, if an elderly patient or a child can't swallow a pill and needs a medication in a liquid form that is not otherwise available, a tasty liquid can be compounded.

All licensed pharmacists learn to perform basic compounding in pharmacy school. The level at which they practice this art varies according to education and desire.

CHAPTER 6

The Hospital
(Too Much Information!)

"Hospital..." – Just *saying* the word can send a chill down the spine. While we are all grateful for hospitals and the services they provide, for most a stay in, or a visit to, one is like stepping into another world....

The World of the ER

Many hospital stays begin in the Emergency Room. But what happens *before* you arrive at the ER *can be life-saving*. Emergency Medical Services (EMS) is a system that provides emergency medical care. EMS providers respond to all kinds of emergencies and hazards, often working side-by-side with police and fire services. *But their primary mission is emergency medical care.*

After a medical emergency as occurred, EMS is activated by calling 9-1-1. The person calling should calmly say what the emergency is. The call-taker will then ask specific questions, in order to dispatch the kind of help that is needed, as quickly as possible.

There are two types of responders specifically trained to provide healthcare in a medical emergency - the EMT (emergency medical technician) and the Paramedic.

Emergency Medical Technicians provide out-of-hospital emergency medical care and transportation for critical and emergent patients who access the EMS system. EMTs have the *basic* knowledge and skills necessary to stabilize and safely transport patients, ranging from non-emergency and medical transports (such as transferring a patient from the hospital back to the nursing home) to life-threatening emergencies. There are two levels of EMTs: EMT-Basic and EMT-Intermediate (also known as an

Advanced EMT). Persons applying for national EMT certification must meet the following requirements:

- 18 years of age or older
- Successful completion of a state-approved EMT course that meets or exceeds the National Emergency Medical Services Education Standards within the past two years
- Have a current CPR-BLS for Healthcare Providers or equivalent certification: *Cardio-Pulmonary Resuscitation- Basic Life Support (CPR-BLS)*. This certification provides training on what to do when someone stops breathing or their heart stops beating, how to use an AED (automatic external defibrillator), and what to do when someone is choking. (*Author's Note*: An AED is a portable device that checks a collapsed person's heart rhythm, and can send an electric shock to the heart to try to restore a normal rhythm. It is used to treat sudden cardiac arrest – when the heart suddenly and unexpectedly stops beating. AEDs are lightweight, battery-operated, and portable devices that are easy to use. Each unit comes with instructions, and the device will even give you voice prompts, telling you what to do. AEDs can be found in places with large numbers of people, such as shopping malls, businesses, airports and airplanes, casinos, convention centers, hotels, sports venues, and schools. You also can purchase an AED for home-use. Both trained and untrained persons can use an AED to help save someone's life)
- Successful completion of the cognitive (knowledge) and a state approved psychomotor (skills) exams

The National Registry of Emergency Medical Technicians (NREMT), an independent, not-for-profit organization, is not a license to practice. But it does validate the competence of certified EMTs. Each state has its own set of rules regarding certification through NREMT and state licensure to practice as an EMT.

The *Paramedic* is an allied health professional who provides *advanced* out-of-hospital emergency medical care for critical and emergent patients who access the EMS. Persons applying for national Paramedic certification must meet the following requirements:

- 18 years of age or older
- Current National Registry certification (NREMT) or state license at the EMT level or higher

- Successful completion of a Commission on Accreditation of Allied Health Education Program (CAAHEP)-accredited Paramedic program within the past two years
- Have a current CPR-BLS for Healthcare Provider or equivalent credential
- Successful completion of the NREMT cognitive (knowledge) and psychomotor (skills) exams

Each state has its own set of rules regarding certification through NREMT and state licensure to practice as a Paramedic.

Communication between the EMS and the Emergency Room is maintained via two-way radio. The ER to which the patient will be transported is notified of the patient's medical condition. When the emergent patient arrives by ambulance, the ER is ready to provide emergency care.

Most often, you, the ill and/or injured patient, will drive yourself to the ER or have someone bring you. Once you arrive, go directly to the reception desk. If you are unable to walk in, the receptionist will have someone assist you in by wheelchair or stretcher. The receptionist will want to know what your medical emergency is (assuming you are conscious and able to provide this), and your pertinent demographic information, including name, address, and insurance. Once this information transfer is complete, you will wait in the waiting room until called. (In the event you are experiencing a life-threatening emergency, you will be taken to be seen right away.)

Once the medical assistant calls out your name, you will be brought back to a holding room or area (known as the *triage*) where more specific questions will be asked and your vital signs taken – blood pressure, temperature, pulse, and respiration rate. A *pulse ox*, a device which is clipped onto your finger, is used to get a quick look of your oxygen level. Additional testing can be done here too, such as labs (blood work), EKG (heart tracing), or an x-ray. An ID bracelet will likely be placed around your wrist.

From the triage room, you may be taken back into the waiting room to wait until you are called, or transported directly back into the Emergency Room. Once you go back into the ER, you may get a room or you may be placed in a hallway until a room is available. Where you go exactly will depend on your illness and the busyness of the ER at the time. If you are temporarily placed in the hallway, you will continue to receive care, just as if you were a patient in a room.

Most Emergency Room patients will experience waiting at some point in time. If it is not a life-threatening emergency, it is helpful for those with you and for you as well, to bring along some sort of entertainment, as well as cell phones and their appropriate electronic chargers. Should you need to make calls to inform others as to what is going on, you will want your phone charged and operational.

The Emergency Room is like no other place. At all hours, you can find a wide variety of medical and ancillary personnel providing services to patients. These personnel include lab technicians, x-ray technicians and their machines, respiratory therapists, Social Services/Care Management, clergy, nursing assistants, and nurses. In addition, there are the medical providers: physicians, nurse practitioners, physician assistants, and a wide variety of specialists. And, should you be in the Emergency Room of a teaching hospital, you will most likely come across Resident and Fellow doctors.

It's important to note the role of teaching hospitals. A *teaching hospital* is a hospital that is affiliated with a medical school, where medical students and Intern, Resident, and Fellow doctors receive clinical training. (Nursing, nurse practitioner, and physician assistant students, as well, may receive part of their training in the hospital setting.)

According to the American Hospital Association, teaching hospitals

- Educate and train future medical professionals
- Conduct state-of-the-art research
- Care for the nation's poor and uninsured people
- Stand ready to provide highly specialized clinical care to the most severely ill and injured

In a teaching hospital, it is common to find Residents and Fellows providing much of the patient care. Know that at each step of the way, these "students", *who have received their Medical Doctor (MD) or Doctor of Osteopath (DO) degree and license,* practice under the guidance of *The Attending,* the senior specialist physician. The Attending oversees all medical decision-making of the Interns, Residents, and Fellows in their respective programs.

It's important for you to know that whether you receive care by a Resident under the direction of The Attending specialist or a non-Resident specialist, it will be of comparable quality.

The Hospital Stay

In the event you are admitted to the hospital, a medical assistant will transport you either by wheelchair or bed to a designated room. But before you leave the Emergency Room, make sure you, your companion, or the medical assistant has gathered up your possessions. Especially important are your eye-glasses, jewelry, and watch, which may have been removed during a procedure. If you do not wish these to go up with you, give them to a trusted loved one for safe-keeping.

Once you are brought to your room, the assistant will help you get transferred into your bed. At this time, the nurse or assistant may ask your family or companions to wait in the hallway in order to respect your privacy. They may take your vital signs again and ask you more questions.

At first, there will be a bit of activity and quite a few personnel in the room. It will be hard for you and your family and friends to know who's who and who's doing what. The RN (registered nurse) will typically wear a bigger badge with "RN" in large letters.

It is common for a white board to be hanging on the wall directly across from your bed. Each shift (this may be eight or twelve hours), the RN and nursing assistant who will be caring for you will have their names written on it, along with the date, so you will know who is caring for you by name.

Keep in mind that many PCPs (primary care providers) do not take care of their patients when they are in the hospital. The *Hospitalist* will do this, communicating with their PCP when needed.

You may or may not have a roommate. While being in a *private* room (you are the only patient) may be preferred, it may not always be an option. In a *semi-private* room, there are two identical side-by-side patient units, separated by a curtain. Each patient room may include a bathroom which may be private (used for that room only) or shared with the patient room on the other side.

Using the Bathroom

Using the bathroom, to urinate and/or to have a bowel movement (poop), can be a challenge for the hospitalized patient. If you need to use the bathroom but are not able or allowed to get out of bed, a *bedpan* is your only option (unless you are a male and can urinate into a urinal). Do not be embarrassed to ask for assistance when using one. Placement is really very important.

If you are able to stand but can't yet walk to the bathroom, a *bedside commode* may be an option for you. This unit is shaped like an arm chair, and has a toilet seat for you to sit on. Underneath the seat is a removable bucket to catch what is eliminated. It can be placed right next to the bed (or wherever is most convenient), allowing for easy transfer.

Many times, it will be necessary for a patient's elimination – what, when, and how much - to be recorded. This information will be written on a log-sheet, which is placed in the room, for documentation by medical personnel. Measuring units and bedpans will be kept in the bathroom. Your bed and room number is written on them to make sure that they will only be used by you.

Should you ever need assistance in using the bathroom, regardless of which method is used, don't hesitate to turn on your call-light. The hospital floor staff is used to assisting patients on and off the bedpan, transferring them onto a bedside commode, and helping them walk to the bathroom. They know how to efficiently manage a patient and any attached IVs, tubes, drains, braces, and/or wires they might have. The last thing anyone wants is for a patient to fall while trying to use the bathroom.

Other things to know about when you are staying in the hospital:

- *Constipation is a common ailment of the hospitalized patient.* Many factors can aggravate this problem, such as decreased or no physical activity, a change in diet, medications, and difficulty getting or avoiding going to the bathroom. Should you begin to experience symptoms of constipation or are prone to being constipated, speak with your RN about having medications available should you need them

- *Blood work is typically drawn in the early morning.* So...expect to be woken up. It is drawn quite early so that when your provider comes in later that morning, your results will be available, and they can make decisions on your plan of care at that time

- *Do not be alarmed by the different smells you may encounter while in a hospital.* Cleanliness and hygiene are a high priority when it comes to the management and control of offensive by-products of illness

- *If, while being a patient, you notice a change in your medical condition, be sure to tell the nurse about it.* It could be an important piece of information not easily identified by your healthcare team

- *The hospital's staff is working at all hours, including during the night.* Sleep may not come easily to you, as it is likely you will hear them moving about. Likewise, the alarms from medical machinery and the response to them may make it difficult to sleep

- *There may be different colored bracelets placed on your wrist if you have medication allergies or special precautions that the staff needs to be aware of.* (For example, the staff needs to know if you have had a *mastectomy* [breast removal], as it is recommended that labs not be drawn on the mastectomy side)

- *Hospital personnel may swipe your ID bracelet on the computer in the room when giving you a medication or performing a procedure, such as drawing blood, to keep track of procedures and expenses*
- *Hand sanitizer is usually available in each room;* you and your visitors should feel free to use it
- *If you are in an Isolation Room due to a contagious illness, those visiting will be required to wear protective equipment.* Hospital staff can assist with the instructions on how to put the equipment on. All visitors, once they return to their homes, should remove the clothing they wore during the visit and wash it. An isolation room may be used to protect you from potential illnesses your visitors may bring, or to protect your visitors from getting your illness
- *The meal tray is for you, the patient. You eat first.* If any leftovers are eaten by family or friends, please let the assistant know when they pick up the tray, as they often record the amount you have eaten. If the assistant writes you ate 100 percent of your meal when you didn't, this can give a false picture of your health to your healthcare team
- *With your (the patient's) permission, family and/or friends may be able to obtain a passcode from the nurse's station that allows them to obtain basic information about your medical condition over the phone*
- *Most likely, you will receive your medications on a different time schedule than when you do at home*
- *Some of the medications you normally take may be substituted with an equivalent type during your hospital stay.* While the hospital pharmacy keeps a wide assortment of medications, keeping a supply of *all* drugs is not practical
- *You are in the hospital because you are sick, so please limit the number and frequency of visitors.* If you are not comfortable telling family and friends to leave, speak with your nurse. They will assist you
- *If you are having trouble understanding what any of your hospital providers have said, ask the nurse*
- *If you have **any** questions, always ask.* Did you receive and understand the results of your test? Why do they want to do another procedure? What is this new medication?
- *If you have insurance, confirm that all providers who participate in your healthcare are in-network.* If you are seen by someone that is not in your insurance

network, you may be billed for services that are not covered by your insurance plan, requiring you to pay out-of-pocket. Just because the hospital you are in is in-network doesn't mean all the providers that work there are

Upon Discharge

Whether you have been discharged from the Emergency Room or from the hospital, you will go home with instructions. This may include bathing or eating instructions, new medication information, wound care, and information regarding follow-up care. These are usually provided by your nurse at the time of your discharge.

The first key piece of information you must follow is to *follow-up*. Most likely, you will be instructed to follow-up with your PCP (primary care provider) within a certain time frame. Or, if you do not have one, a name and contact information may be provided. If you are referred to see a specialist, the hospital staff will provide you with that professional's contact information. However, it is *your* responsibility to schedule the appointment and confirm if they are in-network, for those with insurance.

If you are referred to Specialist A but want to see Specialist B, it may be possible for you to do that. Keep in mind that specialists in a certain field, such as Orthopedics (bone specialist), may not address *all* bone problems. Some may specialize in hips, while others will primarily treat hands. So you may want to contact Specialist B's office to see if they will see you, and if they can take care of your medical problem. If so, and if you have insurance, check to see if Specialist B is in-network.

For those without insurance, shopping around for a specialist can be more difficult. If you were referred to Specialist A when discharged from the hospital and choose to see Specialist A, you may have a better chance of getting an office visit because you were specifically referred there. Tell the receptionist the name of the provider who referred you, and why. Include the specific name of the hospital you were at. Be sure and ask about their self-pay policy. If you want to see a different specialist, you can try contacting someone other than Specialist A and see if they will see you and what the cost will be.

If you need to have a procedure or test done that can wait until after you get home, do your homework:

1. *Do I need to make an appointment with the Specialist, who will be doing the procedure, before having it done?*
   - You may or may not need to schedule an appointment first with the specialist. Contact the specialist's office, using the telephone number

given to you on the discharge papers. They will be able to answer your questions. The answer may depend on whether or not you saw the specialist while in the hospital and the type of procedure you need to have done.

2. *Will my insurance cover the procedure? Do I need a Prior Authorization from my insurance company first?*

   ▪ Per insurance guidelines, certain procedures require a *prior authorization (PA)* from your insurance company before they can be done. Prior Authorization is a process in which your insurance company determines if they will cover a prescribed procedure, service, or medication. The PA process is usually initiated by the ordering provider's office, and requires the filling out of a form detailing why the request is medically necessary. Your insurance company will approve the request, reject it, or request additional information. If it is not authorized, you may be responsible for the total bill.

   ▪ When you first receive the order, speak with the ordering provider's office. Have them confirm that the procedure will be covered by your insurance, before you schedule the appointment. (Document the name of the person you spoke to and when, in the event there is a problem.)

   ▪ Planning ahead assures you that the procedure will be covered and prepares you for any out-of-pocket costs, such as a co-pay or deductible.

3. *Where exactly do I need to go? What entrance should I use?*
4. *Will I need a driver to bring me home? Will I be given a sedative?*
5. *Should I take my prescription medication before the procedure?*
6. *Do I need to be fasting before the procedure and for how long? If I'm not supposed to eat anything, can I drink anything? If yes, what exactly can I drink?*
7. *Will the test or procedure be painful?*
8. *Can I afford it?*

   ▪ Consider price shopping, as not all facilities (e.g., ambulatory surgical and diagnostic centers) charge the same fee for a procedure, such as a *colonoscopy* (a telescope-like instrument that goes up the rectum to look at the large intestines) or an out-patient surgery, such as removal of the gall bladder. Once you find an affordable option, confirm that your provider can do the procedure there. You may even find that prices vary among simpler procedures, such as labs and x-rays (including CT scans, mammograms, and ultrasounds).

- Electronic and Personal Health Record websites and your insurance company's website (if you are insured) may also give you price comparison options. Remember, as long as you have an order, there are options available to you.
- Many of the diagnostic centers and ambulatory surgical centers accept a variety of insurance plans. It never hurts to ask if your insurance is accepted when scheduling a test or procedure.

Another key piece of information you need to take note of upon your hospital discharge will be any *prescriptions*. Any changes to your medication will be printed or written out for you. Remember that the hospital may have substituted some of your medications, such as what you take for high blood pressure. So, question the nurse to determine if whether your discharge hospital medications are going to be treating the same condition as your usual home medications. This is especially important if you are going home with some prescriptions in hand. *You do not want to be taking several pills of the same kind of medication without realizing it, simply because they have different names and appearances!* Once you understand the prescriptions, make sure you get them filled and start them according to the instructions.

Any provider you see for follow-up within the hospital's healthcare system should be able to get information about your hospital stay via the EHR (electronic health record). Still, whether you see a provider in or out of the healthcare system, keep the discharge paperwork together and take it to the follow-up appointment(s). It is better to bring too much information than not enough.

Should you choose or need to see a provider outside of your healthcare system (who may not have access to your EHR,) a *copy of your health record* can be quite helpful. Copies given to, or at least reviewed by your new provider, can help speed up the history-taking process. Be sure to always keep a hard (paper) copy filed away at home for future reference.

You can obtain a hard copy of your medical records in the following ways:

- If you have a PHR and an EHR connected to a healthcare system, you can log into your EHR or PHR website to print the desired records. Usually the clinic or hospital staff automatically adds recent medical activity. You may receive an email notice stating so
- If you do not have a PHR or an EHR, go to the clinic or hospital *Medical Records* department. Once there, you can request the specific medical record(s) you

want. However, to receive the records(s), you will be asked to sign a consent form for the Release of Information (ROI). By signing this form, you give the Medical Records department permission to give you a copy of your health records, as required by the HIPAA privacy act. The department may be able to obtain the information while you wait, or will contact you once the information is ready. Completing your request may take some time, depending on the number and age of the records you have requested. Do not be surprised if there is a fee-per-page charge

When trying to figure what medical records you need, consider the following key pieces of information:

- *Discharge summary*: a chronological summary of your illness history, Emergency Room visit, hospital stay, and discharge instructions
- *Lab reports*: the results of all your blood tests and biopsy reports
- *Radiology reports:* the Radiologist's report is typically all that is needed, which includes x-ray(s), MRI, CT, PET scan, nuclear medicine, and ultrasound. Do not bring the actual films or CD to a follow-up appointment unless requested to do so
- *Medication list*

Essential Know-How about Hospital Bills

For those with insurance, the amount owed for a hospital admission may be very little, or none at all; it depends on the health insurance plan.

For those without insurance, the cost can be devastating. Fortunately, there are ways to minimize the cost of the hospital bill.

Planning ahead for illness is an extremely good first step, although it can be a difficult process to start. Researching health insurance plan options, understanding *terminology* (the meaning of words), and paying the required monthly premiums challenge many people. Finding a good representative who explains the plans and answers your questions is key. (Unfortunately, there is no sure-fire way to find this person.) If at all possible, sit down with the representative versus talking to them over the phone or on the computer. Ask questions, even if you have to ask several times before understanding. If the representative doesn't have the answer, ask to speak with their supervisor. Make notes during your conversation, and highlight key points. Never feel pressured into signing anything. If you need time to think about the options, or want to discuss the plans with someone at home, obtain the contact information for any future questions and who to schedule a follow-up appointment with.

Once you are admitted to the hospital, and you have no or inadequate insurance, you can ask to speak with the *Social Services/Care management* department about payment assistance. This department will be able to answer financial assistance questions and help with the applications for this assistance.

In some circumstances, know that you can decline hospital "extras" that are not medically necessary but will appear on your bill if you receive them. For example, a box of wet wipes (to help with cleaning after using the toilet) may be helpful but not three boxes. Or, ask the nurse if you can bring your own medication from home, as this should be less expensive. However, hospitals have different policies about this practice, so it may or may not be an option.

Once you are discharged, you will most likely be receiving bills from a variety of medical offices and agencies. There is the possibility that you may wish to question the charges of a bill that arrives, so consider following these steps as the bills come in:

1. *Review and organize the bills received.* Your bills may come shortly after your discharge, or they may come months later.
   - Bills from providers may or may not specifically state what date the service was performed, what the service was, and/or who performed the service
   - The Emergency Room and/or hospital bill features a bulk charge. In other words, generally the bill is not itemized or detailed, but includes one charge for all services
   - Each specialist who provided a service to you will send a bill. So there may be bills from providers you have never heard of! For example, if x-rays were reviewed by a Radiologist, a consult was made by an Infectious Disease provider, and anesthesia was needed for a surgery, bills will be sent from the offices of the Radiologist, Infectious Disease provider, and Anesthesiology office. Likewise, if an ambulance was used to get you to the hospital, you can expect a bill from that Business Office
   - If you have insurance, you will receive statements that summarize the charges from all the providers and medical facilities, payments made by your insurance company, prescriptions payments, and the estimate of what is owed by you. This statement is called an *Explanation of Benefits (EOB)*. The EOB typically arrives first, later followed by the bill for payment. (*Author's*

note: Do not pay a bill until you receive a statement that says, "Total due from patient", "Pay this amount", or something similar. You may receive EOBs and statements estimating the amount you owe before the medical claims have been sent through the insurance company and/or are still being processed)

- Always question a bill that arrives after a prolonged amount of time from discharge (greater than one year) or is not consistent with your medical history

2. *Request a detailed bill if it is not itemized.* If you are questioning hospital or ER charges, you will want to ask for a bill that details every single charge individually. This may be called a *"line-item", "itemized", or "detailed"* bill. This will list every single thing you were charged for, large or small. The same can be done if a bill comes through a provider's office.

3. *Keep good notes.* From the very first phone call, write down the date, time, and the name of the person you speak to. Keep legible notes, in case you need to review them months later.

4. *If you find something questionable - something you were billed for and did not receive or a charge you do not understand - begin by handling matters with a phone call.* If you are questioning a bill, whether from a provider or hospital, ask to speak with the Business Office. Again, record the date, time, and agent's name in the event the question is not resolved. This is just the first step, however. Be both persistent and patient, as it may take several steps (phone calls) to complete the process. You even may need to schedule an appointment to meet with the Business Office staff.

5. *Be reasonable with what you are challenging or questioning.* For example, you can't refuse payment simply because you believe the bill to be excessive. When a challenge is made, it must be very specific, such as:
- "I was billed for services I didn't receive," such as an x-ray or a medication
- "I am experiencing double billing for the same service; please check your records."
- "I am being billed for a full-day hospital room rate, but I was discharged in the morning."
- "I see I am being billed for a private room, but I had a semi-private room."
- "It seems I am being charged additional fees on the bill for what are routine supplies, like gowns, gloves, or sheets."

6. *Apply for help within three months of receiving the bill, if you do not have insurance or the resources to pay the bill.* Here are some practical and sometimes quite effective approaches:

- Negotiate with the Business Office about the bill. Before you do so, Internet price-shop the charges among hospitals for comparison. If you discover your hospital is charging more than others, it may give you some leverage
- If the Business Office is unable to help you, ask them who can
- Create a payment plan. Making regular, agreed-upon payments toward your bill may quiet the facility's Business Office
- Ask if the hospital has a financial-assistance program. You may need to be denied for Medicaid before this assistance is approved, however. (*Medicaid* is a government-funded financial assistance for healthcare services for low-income people)
- Consider talking to a medical billing advocate. If your bill is considerable, you might consider paying an advocate, as this may significantly reduce the amount owed. Look for someone who will offer an initial consult free-of-charge. Only after the provider/health facility agrees to a reduced-bill (due to work done by/discussion with the advocate), you pay the advocate a pre-viously agreed-upon amount or a percentage of how much is saved
- Consider alternative fundraising, such as *crowdfunding* - the practice of funding a project or venture by raising many small amounts of money from a large number of people, typically via the Internet through sites like GoFundMe. Donors, often friends and family, can make contributions us-ing their credit cards or through PayPal. If this is something you are inter-ested in doing, be sure and check out the income tax guidelines beforehand

7. *If you have an insurance plan that is declining payment, or you are unable to make payment on what your insurance company didn't pay for, you should*:
    - Keep track of the bills the insurance company rejects on the grounds that the procedure or drug isn't covered by your policy
    - Contact the insurance company to discuss the matter, making sure to always write down whom you spoke to, the phone number, and when (date/time) you spoke to them
    - Challenge the health insurer's decision by requesting an *appeal*. This may require added documentation by the ordering provider
    - Negotiate to see if the insurer will accept the fee assigned to uninsured pa-tients. (Insurance companies privately negotiate contracts and reimburse-ment rates with medical providers and healthcare systems. These contracts determine the "costs" of insured healthcare. With cash-pay patients, costs can be determined by each independent provider or healthcare system)

CHAPTER 7

Preventive (Preventative) Health
(An ounce of prevention is worth a pound of cure - AND dollars!)

*P*revention is vital when it comes to our health. Some things we can change - some things, we cannot. *Heredity*, the genetic make-up we are born with, can't be altered. On the other hand, we *can* choose to make different lifestyle choices, and doing so can greatly influence disease progression.

The keys to halting or impeding disease progression are such healthy lifestyle choices as:

- Lifestyle Key #1: Avoiding behaviors that can cause a health problem
- Lifestyle Key #2: Participating in preventive health opportunities, such as receiving vaccines and screenings for cancer. (These will be discussed in more detail later in this chapter)
- Lifestyle Key #3: Recognizing when there is a problem
- Lifestyle Key #4: Learning everything there is to know about the problem
- Lifestyle Key #5: Making positive changes in behavior to prevent a worsening health situation

Moreover, as a result of decades of medical research, the health industry has introduced to us a host of preventive measures scientifically proven to fight diseases that have documented negative end results (e.g., death, disability, and/or deformity). *Using these measures in conjunction with healthy lifestyle habits and a positive relationship with our PCP is the best combination we can have to cure illness, prevent disease, and promote our own health.* Being proactive like this is a HUGE investment in our health, so let's get started. We'll begin with what many of us receive at the beginning of our lives – vaccines – and then move on to preventive measures for, and screening of, common but serious diseases.

Part A: Vaccines
Vaccines

The most commonly used method for disease prevention is *vaccines* (also known as *immunizations, vaccinations,* and *"baby shots"*). All vaccines used in the U.S. are extensively tested and approved by the U.S. Food and Drug Administration (FDA).

Medical professionals routinely give vaccines to protect their patients from getting certain diseases, and to prevent them from spreading those diseases to others. If a child is exposed to a disease that they have been vaccinated for, the chances of them getting the disease and spreading it to others is *very greatly reduced.*

Vaccines focus on two types of organisms that can cause disease. The first, a *virus,* is a very small, infectious organism that can only live and multiply inside the living cells of other organisms. The second is *bacteria,* single-celled organisms that come in a variety of shapes and are able to live most anywhere. (There are many types of *good bacteria,* with only a few kinds that produce harmful substances and invade tissues, causing infection.)

There are many, many types and combinations of vaccines, with new vaccines and combinations being researched every day. So it is not expected or necessary to know and understand all the names and doses of the various immunizations available. However, having you and your family members regularly seen by your primary care provider for wellness visits, and receiving the recommended vaccines, will go a long ways toward preventing you, your family, and those around you from becoming sick.

If vaccines are used consistently by everyone in a community, it is possible to eliminate diseases that once upon a time debilitated and killed the very young to the very old (e.g., small pox and polio). When a sufficient proportion of community members are immune to a disease (through vaccination and prior illness), the spread of this disease is unlikely. This is called *herd (or community) immunity.* Some protection is even offered to individuals who are not vaccinated (such as newborns and the very ill) because the disease has little opportunity to spread within the community. One of the drawbacks of herd immunity is that people who have the same beliefs about not receiving vaccines frequently live in the same neighborhood, go to the same school, or attend the same religious services. There could be potentially large groups of unvaccinated people living close together. Once the percentage of vaccinated individuals in a population drops below the herd immunity threshold (which can vary among the different diseases), just one exposure to a contagious disease could spread very quickly throughout the community.

For example, let's consider smallpox. *Smallpox* is highly contagious viral illness that causes fever, body aches, and a very distinctive skin rash – raised, pea-sized bumps that open up and drain. While most of the people who have had smallpox recovered, about 30 percent of them died from it. Many smallpox survivors have permanent scars over large areas of their body, and some were left blind. In 1959, the World Health Organization (WHO) initiated a plan to rid the world of smallpox, but it lacked the funds, personnel, and commitment from countries, as well as a shortage of vaccine donations. When the program intensified in 1967, smallpox had been eliminated in North America (1952) and Europe (1953). By 1971 smallpox was eradicated from South America, followed by Asia (1975), and finally Africa (1977). (Smallpox was never widespread in Australia.) *On May 8, 1980, the world was declared free of smallpox, as a direct result of worldwide vaccination.* It is estimated that 300 million people died from smallpox in the 20th century alone. (*Author's note:* Smallpox vaccination ended in the U.S. in 1972. For those readers who received the vaccine, you mostly likely still have the small scar on your upper arm as a result of having received it.)

Traditionally, providers desire to give vaccines to young children because they are the *most defenseless* against certain diseases. Newborn babies are immune to some diseases because they have antibodies (see next paragraph) given to them from their mothers, but this kind of protection only lasts a few months. Furthermore, infants receive no help from their mother's antibodies for diseases such as diphtheria, whooping cough (pertussis), and polio. However, when a healthy baby is born, their immune system is ready to start building a defense to help protect them from disease. There are certain vaccines that can be given to the very young, while others must be given after the baby's immune system has matured with age.

How Vaccines Work

How does a vaccine work? When a vaccine is given, it operates much like an invader trying to attack a city. The invader (the diseased organism in the vaccine) enters a community (the body) and mounts an attack (causing illness). Once the community detects the invasion, a response team (the immune system in the form of *antibodies*) mobilizes to fight the intruder. Each time in the future, when the community (the body) comes into contact with that same invader, the already-organized response team (the body's *antibodies*) quickly fights back, protecting the community from disaster. This immune response, which is produced after receiving a vaccine, can prevent a person from becoming ill with the disease and decreases the risk of spreading it to someone else.

Concerns about Thimerosal

A common concern people have about vaccines revolves around their use of thimerosal. *Thimerosal*, a mercury-based preservative (preservatives kill or prevent growth of bacteria and fungi), was first introduced in 1930. (Its use will be discussed shortly.) It's important to note that there are two types of mercury, which is a naturally-occurring element, found it the earth's crust, air, soil, and water: m*ethylmercury* and *ethylmercury*.

Methylmercury (also known as 'quicksilver') forms when bacteria react with mercury in water, soil, or plants. It can be found in fish swimming in contaminated bodies of water. Because unborn babies are very sensitive to methylmercury's effects, which can cause brain and spinal cord damage, the FDA recommends that women who are pregnant or may become pregnant and nursing mothers should avoid fish that may contain unsafe levels of methylmercury, such as swordfish, king mackerel, shark, and tilefish. (For a list of fish safe and unsafe fish for these women, see www.fda.gov/food/foodborneillnesscontaminants/metals/ucm393070.htm). Methylmercury can also be found in fluorescent lights, batteries, latex paint, and air and water pollution.

Thimerosal contains *ethylmercury*, a preservative that is cleared from the human body more quickly than methylmercury and is less likely to cause harm. In less than one week, one-half of ethylmercury is eliminated from the body, compared to one-half of methylmercury, which takes 1.5 months to eliminate. Ethylmercury is excreted in the intestinal tract, while methylmercury accumulates in the body. When thimerosal enters the body, it breaks down to ethylmercury, which is promptly eliminated.

In 1999, a review of research was published on the effects of thimerosal in childhood vaccines and its relationship with autism. (*Autism* is a complex neurological development disorder identified by repetitive and distinctive patterns of behavior, and difficulties with social communication and interaction. Symptoms present in early childhood.) At that time, the FDA found no evidence of harm, but as a precautionary measure, recommended removing thimerosal from vaccines routinely given to infants.

In 2001, with the exception of some flu vaccines, the Centers for Disease Control (CDC) declared that thimerosal was not to be used as a preservative and was removed from routinely recommended childhood vaccines. With over ten years of research, the CDC has consistently found no association between childhood vaccines and an increased risk of autism.

Thimerosal's purposes are to:

- Prevent contamination during the use of multi-dose vials
- Prevent the growth of bacteria during the vaccine's manufacturing process. However, when thimerosal is used this way, it is removed later in the process, thus leaving only very tiny amounts or none at all behind in the vaccine

Why do we need to use multi-dose vials? To produce enough flu vaccine to immunize the entire U.S. population, for example, some of it must be put into multi-dose vials. Also, multi-dose vials cost less to produce, decrease the amount of medical waste, are easier to distribute, and take up less storage space than using single-dose vials. A multi-dose vial may contain as little as two doses and as many as ten doses. There are many medications that come in both single-dose *and* multi-dose vials. Choosing which option is best is a decision to be made between the patient and their provider.

Each time a new needle is inserted into a multi-dose vial (the top of the vial is cleaned with alcohol and allowed to dry prior to), it is possible for bacteria to get into the vial - and injecting contaminated vaccine into a patient can have tragic consequences. Thimerosal prevents the growth of dangerous bacteria and fungi in these types of vials.

Once opened, all multi-dose vials of medication must be discarded within twenty-eight days, regardless if there is medication still inside, as a precaution against contamination. (When a multi-dose vial is first used, the date it was opened is written on the label.) Also, all vials, regardless if single-use or multi-use, opened or unopened, must be discarded by the expiration date printed on the vial label.

Thimerosal can also be found in eye drops, ear drops, nose sprays, and lotions and skin creams. The preservative actions also prevent bacterial growth in these multi-dose preparations.

Illnesses that Can Be Prevented Through Vaccines

Following is a list of illnesses that can be prevented by using a vaccine designed specifically for that illness. These illnesses are broken down between two types of available vaccine, *live attenuated* and *inactivated* - and the two types of organisms which cause illness, *viruses* and *bacteria*.

A. Live attenuated (weakened) vaccines

These vaccines contain a living organism that is weakened, so it can't actually cause the disease in a person. However, since a live, attenuated vaccine is the closest thing to being exposed to and getting the disease, these vaccines are good "teachers" of the immune system. They often give a person's body lifelong immunity with only one or two doses.

Virus: These viral illnesses can be prevented by using a live attenuated (*weakened*) vaccine:

- *Chicken Pox (varicella)*: a highly contagious disease causing a mild fever and a rash of itchy, inflamed blisters
- *Measles (rubeola)*: a contagious disease causing fever and a red rash on the skin
- *Mumps*: a contagious disease causing swelling of the parotid salivary glands (glands in the mouth that make saliva) and a risk of infertility (inability to have children) in adult males who have had this disease in childhood
- *Rotavirus*: the leading cause of severe gastroenteritis (vomiting and severe diarrhea) among children
- *Rubella (German measles; three-day measles* – which is different from *rubeola measles)*: a contagious disease caused by a virus. The infection is usually mild, with a fever and a rash. However, it can cause deformities in babies if a woman catches it during her pregnancy
- *Shingles (herpes zoster)*: a disease caused by the *varicella virus*, the same virus that causes chickenpox. After a person recovers from chickenpox, the virus quietly rests on a nerve line in the body. For reasons that are not fully known, the virus can *reactivate* (awaken) years later, causing *shingles*, a painful rash that develops along that nerve line on one side of the head or body

- *Smallpox (Vaccinia)*: a serious, contagious, and sometimes fatal infectious disease. The disease is now eliminated after a successful worldwide vaccination program. (The last case of smallpox in the U.S. was in 1949. However, smallpox vaccine is still available in the event of an emergency)

B. *Inactivated (killed) vaccines*

Inactivated vaccines are produced by killing the disease-causing organism with chemicals, heat, or radiation. Because most inactivated vaccines stimulate a weaker immune system response than live (weakened) vaccines, it will likely take several additional doses or *booster shots* to maintain immunity over a lifetime.

Virus: These viral illnesses can be prevented by using an inactivated (*killed*) vaccine:

- *Hepatitis A*: a serious liver disease caused by the hepatitis A virus (HAV). It is found in the stool (poop) of infected people and is usually spread by close personal contact, and sometimes by eating food or drinking water contaminated with HAV
- *Hepatitis B*: a serious disease caused by the hepatitis B virus (HBV) that attacks the liver. The virus can cause a lifelong infection, *cirrhosis* (scarring) of the liver, liver cancer, liver failure, and death. It is spread through contact with infected blood and body fluids, such as saliva, semen, and vaginal secretions. The hepatitis B vaccine involves a series of three shots given at different times. It can cause a burning sensation when injected into the muscle. (*Author's Note*: There is no need to restart the series of three shots, even if years have passed between your receiving the shots. Simply begin where you left off)
- *Human Papillomavirus (HPV)*: a common virus spread through sexual contact. (It is considered a Sexually Transmitted Disease/Infection – STD/I.) HPV can cause cervical (cervix) cancer in women, cancer in both men and women (genital, head and neck), and genital warts in both men and women. The HPV vaccine works by preventing the most common types of HPV from causing cervical cancer and genital warts. Research is in progress to see if the vaccine will also prevent head and neck cancers caused by HPV
- *Influenza (flu)*: a contagious respiratory illness caused by influenza viruses that can cause mild to severe illness. The serious outcomes of flu infection can result in hospitalization or death. There are three types of flu virus: A, B, and C. Influenza

A and B cause seasonal epidemics of disease nearly every winter. Type C infections cause mild respiratory illnesses, and are not thought to cause epidemics. For those readers who are interested in a more scientific study of the influenza vaccine, check out the following points:

a. Influenza A is divided into subtypes based on two proteins found on the surface of the virus: hemagglutinin (H) has 18 subtypes, and neuraminidase (N), which has 11 subtypes.

b. Influenza B viruses are not divided into subtypes, but they can be further broken down into lineage and strain.

The Centers for Disease Control and Prevention (CDC) follow an internationally accepted naming process for influenza viruses:

- The antigenic type (A, B, C)
- The host of origin, for example swine or chicken. *For human-origin viruses, no host of origin designation is given*
- Geographical origin
- Strain number
- Year of isolation
- For influenza A viruses, the H and N description

For example, for the influenza season of 2015 (fall) -2016 (spring), the flu vaccine contained

- A/California/7/2009 (H1N1) virus
- A/Switzerland/9715293/2013 (H3N2) virus
- B/Phuket/3073/2013 virus

The 2016-2017 flu vaccine contained

- A/California/7/2009 (H1N1)-like virus
- A/Hong Kong/4801/2014 (H3N2)-like virus
- B/Brisbane/60/2008-like virus (B/Victoria lineage)

The 2017-2018 flu vaccine contains

- A/Michigan/45/2015 (H1N1)pdm09-like virus

- A/Hong Kong/4801/2014 (H3N2)-like virus
- B/Brisbane/60/2008-like virus (B/Victoria lineage)

An Avian (bird) flu example is: A/duck/Hong Kong/147/77(H9N6).

Flu vaccine is made three different ways. Two of the processes are egg-based. The third process, called *recombinant*, does not use eggs, and thus can be used for those who are allergic to eggs.

The flu viruses selected each year for the flu vaccine are based on the findings of 142 influenza centers around the world researching flu virus trends, such as which flu viruses are circulating, how the viruses are spreading, and how well current vaccine ingredients are protecting against newly identified viruses. The standard flu vaccine contains three strains of flu virus, whereas the *high-dose* flu vaccine contains 4 strains. The high-dose flu vaccine is recommended for those sixty five years and older because the immune system weakens with age, which places them at greater risk of severe illness from the flu. A higher dose gives older people a better immune response, and therefore, better protection against the flu.

Flu viruses are constantly changing and mutating in a process called *antigenic drift*. These are small changes in the genes of influenza viruses that happen continually over time as the virus replicates. Because of these changes, your immune system can't recognize the flu virus from year to year. That is why you need to get a new flu vaccine each year.

- Polio: a crippling and potentially deadly infectious disease caused by a virus that lives in the throat and intestinal tract. It is spread through person-to-person contact with the stool of an infected person, or through nose and mouth secretions. Polio virus can invade an infected person's brain and spinal cord, causing paralysis in parts of the body. The U.S. stopped using live oral polio vaccine in 2000 due to an increased risk of vaccine-associated paralytic polio. (Worldwide, polio cases have decreased by over 99% since 1988, from an estimated 350 000 cases then, to 37 reported cases in 2016. As a result of the global effort to eradicate the disease through vaccination, more than 16 million people have been saved from paralysis)
- Rabies: a disease transmitted through the bite of an animal infected with rabies. The virus infects the central nervous system (brain and spinal cord), ultimately causing disease in the brain and death. The rabies virus is transmitted through saliva or brain/nervous system tissue. A person (or

animal) can only get rabies by coming in contact with bodily excretions and tissues

Bacteria: These bacterial illnesses can be prevented by using an inactivated (*killed*) vaccine:

- *Diphtheria*: a serious, possible fatal disease. It causes a thick coating in the back of the nose or throat that makes it hard to breathe or swallow
- *Haemophilus influenza B* (Hib): a cause of bacterial infections that is often severe, particularly among infants. The vaccine prevents *meningitis* (an infection of the covering of the brain and spinal cord), *pneumonia* (lung infection), *epiglottitis* (a severe throat infection), and other serious infections
- *Meningococcal disease*: a serious illness that is a leading cause of bacterial meningitis (see previous entry) in children two through eighteen years old in the U.S. Serogroups A, B, C, W, and Y are responsible for most cases of meningitis. (There are two vaccines available: A, C, W, Y combination and B. *See below*)
- *Pertussis (whooping cough)*: a highly contagious respiratory disease. Pertussis is known for its uncontrollable, violent coughing, which can make it hard to breathe - resulting in a *"whooping"* sound. Pertussis most commonly affects infants and young children, and can be fatal, especially in babies less than one year of age
- *Pneumococcal disease*: a very serious bacterial infection that causes pneumonia, meningitis, and infection in the blood
- *Tetanus (lockjaw)*: a serious bacterial disease that causes painful tightening of the muscles, usually all over the body. It can lead to a *"locking"* of the jaw so the patient cannot open their mouth or swallow. The bacteria that cause tetanus are found in soil. They get into the body through a puncture, cut, or sore on the skin. A person can also become infected after a burn or an animal bite

Routine Vaccines

Following is a listing of illnesses that people are routinely vaccinated for, along with the vaccine given. The first grouping is for children, newborn to eighteen years of age. The second grouping is for adults, eighteen years of age to the elderly. Listed next to the vaccine is the link to the CDC's Vaccine Information Statement (VIS). The CDC's vaccine information statements explain:

- what the vaccine does,
- who should get the vaccine, and
- what the side effects are.

For each age group, I have included a link to an easy-to-read chart of recommended vaccines.

Author's Note: When considering you and your family's medical history, and the multiple combinations of vaccines, it is advisable that you discuss with your provider or local health department what vaccines are recommended specifically for you and your family members.

Childhood (newborn through eighteen years of age):
www.cdc.gov/vaccines/schedules/easy-to-read/index.html

1. Diphtheria, Tetanus, acellular Pertussis: DTaP (A tetanus shot, in any combination, can make the muscle quite sore for both the young and old; *Acellular* means only pieces of a pertussis cell are used, not the whole cell – which, in earlier vaccines, caused more side effects)
   www.cdc.gov/vaccines/hcp/vis/vis-statements/dtap.html
2. *Haemophilus influenza* type b (Hib):
   www.cdc.gov/vaccines/hcp/vis/vis-statements/Hib.html
3. Hepatitis A: HAV, Hep A
   www.cdc.gov/vaccines/hcp/vis/vis-statements/hep-a.html
4. Hepatitis B: HBV, Hep B
   www.cdc.gov/vaccines/hcp/vis/vis-statements/hep-b.html
5. Human Papillomavirus (HPV)
   www.cdc.gov/vaccines/hcp/vis/vis-statements/hpv-gardasil-9.html
6. Influenza (Flu)
   www.cdc.gov/vaccines/hcp/vis/vis-statements/flu.html
7. Measles, Mumps, Rubella: MMR
   www.cdc.gov/vaccines/hcp/vis/vis-statements/mmr.html
8. Meningococcal: MCV
   - A, C, W, Y: www.cdc.gov/vaccines/hcp/vis/vis-statements/mening.html
   - B: www.cdc.gov/vaccines/hcp/vis/vis-statements/mening-serogroup.html

9. Pneumococcal: PCV
    - *Prevnar 13[R]*: www.cdc.gov/vaccines/hcp/vis/vis-statements/pcv13.html
    - *Pneumovax[R]*: www.cdc.gov/vaccines/hcp/vis/vis-statements/ppv.html
10. Polio: IPV (Inactivated Polio Vaccine)
    www.cdc.gov/vaccines/hcp/vis/vis-statements/ipv.html
11. Rotavirus: RV
    www.cdc.gov/vaccines/hcp/vis/vis-statements/rotavirus.html
12. Tdap: Tetanus, diphtheria, acellular pertussis: Booster shot (This vaccine contains the same components as the infant-childhood vaccine, DTaP, and is given to boost immunity – a *"booster"* shot)
    www.cdc.gov/vaccines/hcp/vis/vis-statements/tdap.html
13. Varicella (chicken pox)
    www.cdc.gov/vaccines/hcp/vis/vis-statements/varicella.html

Adult (nineteen years of age and older):
www.cdc.gov/vaccines/schedules/easy-to-read/index.html

1. Hepatitis A: HAV, Hep A
    www.cdc.gov/vaccines/hcp/vis/vis-statements/hep-a.html
2. Hepatitis B: HBV, Hep B
    www.cdc.gov/vaccines/hcp/vis/vis-statements/hep-b.html
3. HPV (Human Papillomavirus)
    www.cdc.gov/vaccines/hcp/vis/vis-statements/hpv-gardasil-9.html
4. Influenza (Flu)
    www.cdc.gov/vaccines/hcp/vis/vis-statements/flu.html
5. Measles, Mumps, Rubella: MMR
    www.cdc.gov/vaccines/hcp/vis/vis-statements/mmr.html
6. Meningococcal: MCV
    - A, C, W, Y: www.cdc.gov/vaccines/hcp/vis/vis-statements/mening.html
    - B: www.cdc.gov/vaccines/hcp/vis/vis-statements/mening-serogroup.html
7. Pneumococcal: PCV
    - *Prevnar13[R]*: www.cdc.gov/vaccines/hcp/vis/vis-statements/pcv13.html
    - *Pneumovax[R]*: www.cdc.gov/vaccines/hcp/vis/vis-statements/ppv.html

8. Tetanus, diphtheria, acellular pertussis: Booster shot (This vaccine contains the same components as the infant childhood vaccine, DTaP, and is given to boost immunity – a "*booster*" shot)
   - Tdap: www.cdc.gov/vaccines/hcp/vis/vis-statements/tdap.html
   - Td: www.cdc.gov/vaccines/hcp/vis/vis-statements/td.html
9. Varicella (chicken pox)
   www.cdc.gov/vaccines/hcp/vis/vis-statements/varicella.html
10. Zoster Vaccine (Shingles)
    www.cdc.gov/vaccines/hcp/vis/vis-statements/varicella.html

Author's Note: As of this writing, *needle-free injection*, a way of giving shots without using a needle, is beginning to become available. It is used in a handful of medications, including insulin, *Epipen*[R], and one type of flu vaccine. The device works by forcing a medication (powder or liquid) through the skin at a high rate of speed. While the advantages of using such a system with vaccines are many, the technology is still quite complex and expensive. There are currently three types of needle-free injection methods: spring-loaded, battery-powered, and gas-powered.

Part B: Preventive Measures for Common Diseases and Conditions
Osteoporosis Screening

Our bones are made of living tissues that change in each cycle of our lives. Even after we stop growing, our bones continue to become denser. Peak bone mass (the amount of bone tissue) is reached up to 90 percent by age eighteen in girls, and by age twenty in boys. During this time, we are making more bone than losing bone mass. Our bones continue to increase in density until age thirty, when they are at their strongest.

All bones are made the same. The hard outer part, the *cortical bone*, is largely made of *proteins* (collagen) and *hydroxyapatite* (calcium and other minerals). Hydroxyapatite is mainly responsible for the strength and density of bones. Our bones also are covered by a thin layer called the *periosteum*, where pain-sensing nerves are located. Blood enters the bones through blood vessels that enter through the periosteum.

The inner part of bones, the *trabecular bone*, is softer and less dense than the hard outer part, but still plays a large part in bone strength. Reducing the amount or quality of trabecular bone increases the risk of fractures, such as with aging or bone disease. *Bone marrow* is the living tissue that fills the spaces in the trabecular bone.

Bones have two shapes - *flat*, such as the plates of the skull and sternum (breastbone) - and *tubular*, such as the finger or leg bones.

Our bones have many purposes:

- Serve as our supporting framework
- Allow for movement
- Protect our internal organs. For example, our skull bones protect our brain, the breastbone (*sternum*) and ribcage protect our heart and lungs, and our back bones (*vertebrae*) protect our spinal nerves
- Store calcium and phosphorus, which keeps our bones strong, and releases them when our bodies need them for other purposes
- The bone marrow makes *red blood cells* (responsible for carrying oxygen), *white blood cells* (responsible for fighting infection, e.g., through the immune system), and *platelets* (responsible for our blood clotting, such as after being cut)

Our bones are continually changing in a process called *remodeling*. During this process, small areas of old bone are removed and gradually replaced by new bone. It is a continuous process, with every bone in our body completely reformed about every ten years.

To keep our bones dense and strong, we need an adequate supply of calcium, vitamin D, and other minerals. Our young bodies also produce the necessary amounts of several hormones, such as estrogen, testosterone, parathyroid hormone, and growth hormone, which help to keep our bones strong. Weight-bearing activity, such as walking, also helps to strengthen bones.

Once we reach middle age, bone loss tends to speed up. This is especially true for women, once they reach *menopause* (the "change of life", when menstrual periods stop). The hormone *estrogen* plays a large and important part in maintaining strong bones. However, after menopause, there is less estrogen made, leading to greater bone loss. A woman can lose up to 20 percent or more of her bone density after menopause.

Osteoporosis, meaning *"porous bone,"* happens when we lose too much bone, do not make enough bone, or both. The result is weaker bones that can easily break. Osteoporosis is caused by both genetic (e.g., heredity, and the things we can't change about ourselves) and environmental (things that we can change) factors.

Risk Factors for Osteoporosis:

1. **Genetics**
    -   Gender: Women get osteoporosis more often than men
    -   Age: The older we are, the greater our risk of osteoporosis
    -   Body size: Small frame. Thin women are at greater risk
    -   Ethnicity: White and Asian women are at highest risk. African-American and Hispanic women have a lower risk
    -   Family history: Osteoporosis tends to run in families. If a family member has osteoporosis or breaks a bone, there is a greater chance that we will too
    -   Women: Low estrogen levels due to menopause
    -   Men: Low testosterone
2. **Environmental**
    -   An eating disorder called *anorexia nervosa*, which makes people lose more weight than is considered healthy for their age and height
    -   Low diet intake of calcium and vitamin D
    -   Some medications
    -   Lack of exercise
    -   Smoking
    -   Drinking alcohol

The best test to determine your current bone health is called a *Bone Mineral Density* (BMD, DXA, DEXA) test. This test compares your bones to that of a thirty year old. (Remember, this is the age at which your bones are the strongest.) The BMD test is quick and painless, and is very much like having an x-ray taken. It usually requires an order from your provider, which you will need to take with you.

It is recommended you not take any vitamins, supplements, or antacids containing calcium twenty-four hours before your test, as it can interfere with the BMD results. You may be asked to change into a gown. Any metal objects, such as zippers, keys, and belts, may need to be removed. If you have had a recent test requiring barium or an injected contrast (dye) material, you must wait ten to fourteen days before having a BMD test. Inform the technician if you are pregnant.

Here are the guidelines as to who should get an osteoporosis screening.

Guidelines for Osteoporosis Screening

1. U. S. Preventive Services Task Force (USPSTF: an independent, volunteer panel of national experts in prevention and evidence-based medicine): www.uspreventiveservicestaskforce.org/Page/Topic/recommendation-summary/osteoporosis-screening
   a. *BMD screening recommendations for women*:
      - Women aged sixty-five years and older
      - Women younger than sixty-five years with risk factors similar to that of a white, sixty-five year old woman (see previous)
   b. *BMD screening recommendations for men*:
      - Current evidence is insufficient to assess the balance of benefits and harms of screening for osteoporosis in men, (meaning there is not enough evidence to show the screening is helpful or harmful)

   (Author's note: As of this writing, this topic is in the process of being updated by the USPSTF)
2. National Osteoporosis Foundation: nof.org/articles/743
   a. *BMD screening recommendations for women*:
      - Women aged sixty-five or older
      - women of menopausal age with risk factors (see previous)
      - women under age sixty-five with risk factors (see previous)
      - women who break a bone after age fifty
   b. *BMD screening recommendations for men*:
      - Men aged seventy and older
      - men aged fifty through sixty-nine with risk factors (see previous)
      - men who break a bone after age fifty

If having the screening is advisable for you, your provider can give you the order and instruct you as to where you can get a BMD test done. Taking this screening test falls under "Preventive Health", and is usually covered by insurance plans (if you have one). Usually the screening is done every two years, based on your risk factors and diagnosis. The resulting number of the BMD test is called the *T-score*:

- A T-score of 0 (zero) means you have the bones of a healthy thirty year old ("Normal" is +1 to -1)
- A T-score of -1 to -2.5 means you have low bone mass or bone-thinning, also called *osteopenia*. Here, your bone mass falls between normal and osteoporosis
- A T-score of -2.5 or lower gives you a diagnosis of osteoporosis. This happens when you lose too much bone, make too little bone, or both. As a result, your bones become weak or fragile, and may easily break

Cancer Screening

There are very few people who have not been affected by cancer in one way or another. While there are many causes to be considered, they basically can be boiled down to these two factors - genetics and environmental. Genetics, as previously mentioned, cannot be altered. However, you can alter your environment, through the everyday choices you make, and in turn this can positively affect your health and well-being.

Being proactive by taking cancer screenings is a form of Preventive Health. Detecting a cancer before symptoms appear can greatly improve the treatment outcome and a person's quality of life. So carefully consider the screenings discussed below. Then talk with your primary care provider about what is advisable for you based on your personal health history and risk factors.

Breast Cancer

A. Breast Self-Exam

This author recommends that every adult woman and man be familiar with their breasts. The American Cancer Society estimates that in 2017, about 252,710 new cases of breast cancer will be diagnosed in women, and cause about 40,610 deaths. There will be about 2,470 men diagnosed with breast cancer, and 460 men will die from it.

Conducting a monthly *self-breast exam* helps you in finding an abnormality that may not have previously been there. To better remember that you need to do regular breast exams, plan to do your exam on the first day of each month, after your period has started, or when starting a new pack of birth control pills, for example. Report any changes to your PCP or Gynecologist (female specialist). Changes you need to look for include:

- A mass that is painless, hard, and has irregular edges. This type of mass is more likely to be cancerous, although some breast cancers can be tender, soft, or rounded
- Swelling of all or part of a breast, even if no distinct lump is felt
- Skin irritation or dimples
- Breast or nipple pain
- A nipple that is turning inward, like it's being pulled inside
- Redness, scaling, or thickening of the nipple or breast skin
- Any nipple discharge (other than breast milk)

How to Do a Breast Self-Exam
Stand in front of a mirror: *Looking*

1. Look closely at your nipples, the *areola* (dark part around the nipple), and the skin of your breast from your collarbone to the top of your abdomen, and from your armpit to your breastbone. Here's what you should look for:
   - Breasts that are their usual size, shape, and color
   - Breasts that are evenly shaped without swelling or deformed appearance
   - Dimples, puckers, skin bulges, redness, crusting, or rash
   - Any signs of fluid coming out of one or both nipples. This discharge may be watery, milky, yellowish, or bloody
2. Place your hands on your hips and push. While doing this, look at your chest for any abnormalities between the tightened chest wall muscles and skin
3. Raise your arms over your head, place your hands behind your head, and lean forward. Look again for the same changes

Lay down flat on your back: *Feeling*

1. Place the arm of the side of the breast to be checked under your head. (Doing so spreads out the breast tissue evenly over the chest wall and also thins the breast, making it much easier to feel all the breast tissue. For women with

large breasts, it may be helpful to place a small pillow under that side of your back to help roll the breast tissue onto your chest.)

2. Using quarter-sized, circular motions of the three middle finger pads of the opposite hand, move your fingers around the breast in an up-and-down pattern. Begin at an imaginary line drawn straight down your side from the underarm, and move across the breast to the middle of the breast bone in an up-and-down pattern. Be sure to check the entire breast area, going down until you feel only ribs and up to the neck or collar bone.

3. As you move your fingers around the breast, be sure to use three different levels of pressure to feel all the breast tissue: *Light pressure* to feel the tissue closest to the skin; *medium pressure* to feel a little deeper; and *firm pressure* to feel the tissue closest to the chest and ribs. Note: It is normal to feel a firm ridge in the lower curve of each breast.

4. Repeat steps the previous three steps on the other breast.

At well-woman exams, either your PCP or your gynecologist may perform a *clinical breast exam* (CBE), which is a breast exam performed by a healthcare provider.

B. Mammogram

A *mammogram* is an x-ray of the breast. Its purpose is to detect and evaluate changes in the breast tissue. There are two types of mammogram:

- A *screening mammogram* is done when you are having no breast problems or signs of cancer. Its purpose is to detect abnormalities that can't be seen or felt. Two views of each breast are taken - top to bottom and sideways. (For larger breasts, more than two x-rays may be taken)
- A *diagnostic mammogram* is done when a problem has been found in the breast, such as a lump or an abnormality in the screening mammogram. Additional x-rays will be taken, allowing the technologist to magnify the area of concern for a closer look

What happens during the mammogram?

During the mammogram, the breast is briefly compressed between two plates attached to the mammogram machine. There is an adjustable top plate that is clear and a fixed bottom plate. The bottom plate holds the x-ray film that records the image.

Before taking the image, the technologist compresses the breast between the upper and lower plates to keep it from moving, and to make the layer of breast tissue thinner. The thinner the breast layer is, the better the x-ray picture will be. *Compression*, or flattening, of the breast is important because it spreads the breast tissue out so those reading the mammogram can see details of the tissue more clearly. It also reduces the amount of radiation you will receive during the procedure, as well as any breathing motion during the x-ray.

Although the compression during a mammogram can feel uncomfortable, even painful, it is needed to get a good picture - and it lasts only *a few seconds*. If you find it is too painful, you can always talk to your technologist. She may be able to reposition you to make enduring the pressure more comfortable for you.

For women with larger breasts, the technologist may need to use a larger plate or possibly more than one plate to get good views of all the breast tissue.

A newer form of mammogram testing, called *breast tomosynthesis or 3-D mammography*, is available as of this writing. For this test, a machine takes many low-dose x-ray images as it moves over the breast. The images are recorded onto a computer, which combine them into a three-dimensional picture. Three-D mammography uses more radiation than most standard two-view mammograms, but it may let doctors see problem areas more clearly.

For women who have implants, the x-rays used for imaging the breasts cannot penetrate silicone or saline implants well enough to show the breast tissue that is over or under it. This means that the part of the breast tissue covered up by the implant will not be seen on the mammogram. In order that the technologist and Radiologist see as much breast tissue as possible, women with implants have four additional pictures as well as the four standard pictures taken during the screening mammogram. For these extra x-ray pictures, implants that are placed *over* the chest wall muscle are pushed back against the chest wall, and the breast is pulled forward over it. This allows better imaging of the front part of each breast. Implant views can be quite difficult to obtain from (and uncomfortable) for those women who have hardened scar tissue formation around the implants. Generally, it is easier to obtain implant views in women whose implants are placed *underneath* (behind) the chest wall muscle.

Paying for a Mammogram

A common factor that affects the decision on whether or not a woman gets a mammogram is money. If you have insurance, a screening mammogram is usually covered under "Preventive Health" services, and there is no cost. If a diagnostic mammogram is ordered (meaning an abnormality has been identified), a diagnosis is made and a claim will be filed with your insurance company after the mammogram is taken. This is where a deductible and/or co-payment may come into play. There will be a diagnostic mammogram bill from the diagnostic center, plus a bill from the Radiologist who reads the x-ray.

For those without insurance, there are options. Consider scheduling your mammogram in October, which is Breast Cancer month, as many diagnostic facilities offer reduced mammogram fees during this month. Or, call ahead of time to schedule your mammogram; this allows you to do some financial planning when it comes to payment. You can call different diagnostic centers and shop around for the best price. Also, watch for healthcare systems' advertisements in local newspapers that may indicate if there are any reduced fees for mammograms throughout the year.

The Centers for Disease Control (CDC) sponsors the National Breast and Cervical Cancer Early Detection Program (NBCCEDP), which provides access to breast and cervical cancer screening services to underserved women in all fifty states, the District of Columbia, five U.S. territories, and eleven tribes. This service supports programs that offer clinical breast examinations, mammograms, and referrals for treatment. You may be eligible for a free or low-cost mammogram if you meet the following qualifications:

- Between forty and sixty-four years of age for breast cancer screening
- Have no insurance, or have insurance that does not cover screening exams
- Your yearly income is at or below 250 percent of the federal poverty level

Information about the NBCCEDP can be obtained by calling the Centers for Disease Control and Prevention (CDC) at 800-232-4636 or at their website: www.cdc.gov/cancer/nbccedp/about.htm. The American Cancer Society may also be helpful in finding low cost or free mammograms in your area if you do not meet the criteria for the NBCCEDP. Their telephone number is 800- 227-2345.

The Mammogram Appointment

Talk to your PCP, staff at your local hospital, or a friend to help locate a mammogram facility near you. Also, check your insurance website for covered options. Many times a mammogram facility is located in a diagnostic center, where other kinds of testing can be done, such as lab, x-ray, and bone mineral density tests.

When you call to make an appointment, the receptionist will ask you questions, such as your name, date of birth, and insurance information. They may verify you have an order from your provider, as many facilities require one to do the test. If so, bring this order in with you when you have your mammogram done. When making your appointment, choose a date when your breasts will not be sore or sensitive, something which is common before your menstrual period begins.

If you are going to a mammogram facility that you've not been to previously, it is helpful to bring a list of places and dates of any previous mammograms, biopsy information, or other breast treatments received. If you had a previous mammogram(s) done at a different facility, the diagnostic center will request their contact information and may have you sign a Release of Information (ROI) to obtain the earlier x-ray films for comparison. Viewing the old and new mammograms side by side allows the Radiologist to compare areas of concern – e.g., if it is a new change, or has not changed from previous x-rays. However, it can take up to two weeks to receive the films, which may delay the final reading of your mammogram. So having the name and address of where the previous mammograms were performed will quicken the process. When calling to schedule, the receptionist may also ask for this information, allowing them to obtain the previous films prior to your arrival.

Once you arrive for a mammogram, you may be escorted to a changing area. It is helpful to wear a skirt or pants to the appointment, so all that you will need to remove is your top and bra. Be sure to remove any jewelry that may interfere with the x-ray, such as a necklace or dangling earrings.

Importantly, the attendant will ask you to remove any underarm deodorant, lotions, or powder. Particles from deodorant and/or powder can resemble micro-calcifications on the x-ray. *Micro-calcifications*, small calcium deposits that look like white specks on a mammogram, can be a sign of breast cancer. In the changing area you may find wipes for your underarms.

To get ready, you will have to undress from the waist up and put on a gown. A locker with a key may be available for you to place your personal items. If not, be prepared to take your purse and clothing with you. Then you will sit and wait in a private waiting room until it is your turn.

The technologist will escort you to the mammogram room, where it will only be the two of you in the room. They will take a brief history, and ask questions, such as:

- What is your date of birth?
- Do you have any family or personal history of breast cancer?
- Are you experiencing any breast problems?
- Have you had a mammogram before?

- Do you have breast implants?
- Are you pregnant or breastfeeding?

Then they will take the x-rays, with the technologist instructing you each step of the way. Know that she will handle your breasts to get them into the best possible position. She also will advise you on arm and body placement. It will be necessary for your chest wall to come up against the mammogram machine and your arm lifted up out of the way. Relax your upper body and chest wall muscles as much as possible to ease the process.

It may be helpful to focus on an object away from your breast during compression, or count as a distraction. It is also very important to try not to breathe during image-taking, as movement on your part can create a blurry picture. So the technologist will tell you when to hold your breath, and when to start breathing normally again.

A screening mammogram takes fifteen to twenty minutes in total, while the actual breast compression lasts only a few seconds each time. Once the technologist has confirmed the images are of good quality, she will escort you back to the changing room, and a Radiologist will read your x-rays. You may be given the option to wait for the results, or be given a phone number to call later that day for results. Either way, you and the provider who wrote the order will receive a report in the mail or electronically.

If you receive an abnormal report, a diagnostic mammogram will most likely be ordered. If the diagnostic mammogram is abnormal, a breast ultrasound and possibly a biopsy will follow.

Risk Factors for Breast Cancer:

1. **Genetic**
   - Being female: Breast cancer is one hundred times more common in women than men
   - Age: Two-thirds of women are diagnosed with breast cancer after age fifty-five. About one out of eight breast cancers are found in women younger than forty-five
   - White
   - Family History: Mother, sister, father, child. There's an increased risk if the family member is diagnosed before age fifty
   - Have had breast cancer in one breast
   - Periods began before age twelve, started menopause after age fifty-five, had your first child after the age thirty, and/or have never given birth

- Genetic mutations/heredity, such as gene BRCA1 and BRCA2 (BRCA = BReast CAncer)
- Dense breast tissue (female hormones play an important role in the density of breast tissue)

2. **Environmental**
   - Lack of physical activity
   - Poor diet: Diet high in saturated fat and lacking fruits and vegetables
   - Being overweight or obese
   - Drinking alcohol: The more alcohol you consume, the greater the risk
   - Radiation to the chest before the age of thirty
   - Combined hormone replacement therapy (HRT): Taking combined hormone replacement therapy (estrogen and progestin) for menopause symptoms can increase your risk

Guidelines for Breast Cancer Screening for Women of Average Risk
Women of average risk are considered to be those who

- are having no breast symptoms
- have not been previously diagnosed with breast cancer
- are not at high-risk for getting breast cancer as a result of an underlying genetic mutation
- have no history of chest radiation at a young age

In terms of the recommended guidelines for breast cancer screening, there are two main trains of thought. Bear in mind these organizations' recommendations are intended for women who are *not* at increased risk of developing breast cancer, and so only apply to *routine* screening procedures. As always, it is vital that you have a conversation with your PCP about what is recommended specifically for *you*. Also, please note that although women with implants do have more pictures taken at each mammogram, the guidelines for how often women with implants should have screening mammograms are the same as for women without them.

1. U. S. Preventive Services Task Force (USPSTF): www.uspreventiveservices taskforce.org/Page/Document/UpdateSummaryFinal/breast-cancer-screening1?ds=1&s=breast%20cancer%20screening
   a. *Breast Self-Exam*: No recommendation

    b.   *Clinical Breast Exam*: No recommendation

    c.   *Mammography*:

- Women before age fifty: Decision is based on the patient's personal medical history (present and past), patient preference, and family history
- Women fifty through seventy-four years: Every two years
- Women seventy-five years and older: There is not enough evidence showing whether screening is helpful or not

4.   American Cancer Society: www.cancer.org/healthy/findcancerearly/cancerscreeningguidelines/chronological-history-of-acs-recommendations

    a.   *Breast Self-Exam*: Women twenty and older: Optional.

Women should be told about the benefits and limitations of breast self-exams. They should report any new symptoms to their healthcare provider

    b.   *Clinical Breast Exam*:

- Women ages twenty through thirty-nine years: Part of a periodic health exam, preferably every three years
- Women ages forty years and older: Part of a periodic health exam, preferably every year

    c.   *Mammography*:

- Women ages forty through forty-four: Women in this age group should have the choice to start annual screening with mammograms if they wish to do so. The risks of screening as well as the potential benefits should be considered in conjunction with a PCP or Gynecologist (*see below*)
- Women ages forty-five through fifty five: Yearly
- Women ages fifty-five and older: Every two years. Women should also have the chance to continue yearly screening if they choose to. The screening mammograms should continue as long as a woman is in good health and is expected to live at least ten more years

There has been some controversy on whether having a mammogram is more harmful than not having one. The decision to have a mammogram is between you and your provider. Many factors will be considered, such as your personal health history, your risk factors, and the health history of your family members.

Early detection of breast cancer with screening mammography means that treatment can be started earlier in the course of the disease, possibly before it has spread. Research results show that screening mammography can help reduce the number of deaths from breast cancer among women ages forty to seventy-four, especially for those over age fifty. Studies have not shown a benefit from regular screening mammography in women under the age of forty.

The benefits of screening mammography need to be balanced against its harms, which include:

1. *Radiation exposure*:
   - Radiation dose is very low
   - Repeated x-rays can increase the risk of cancer
2. *False-Positive results*: Occurs when the Radiologist sees an abnormality on the mammogram when no cancer is present
   - Additional testing is done to determine if cancer is present. A diagnostic mammogram, breast ultrasound, and/or biopsy can be costly, time consuming, and physically uncomfortable
   - Can lead to anxiety and psychological distress
   - Are more common in younger women, women with dense breasts, women who have had a previous breast biopsy, a family history of breast cancer, and women who are taking estrogen
3. *False-Negative results*: Occurs when no abnormality is identified on the mammogram even though breast cancer is present
   - Screening mammograms miss about 20 percent of breast cancers
   - Occur more often in women with dense breast tissue and younger women
   - Can lead to delays in treatment
   - May give women a false sense of security
4. *Over-diagnosis and Over-treatment*:
   - Screening mammograms can find breast cancers and cases of ductal carcinoma in situ (DCIS) that need to be treated. (DCIS: a build-up of abnormal cells in the lining of breast ducts that *may* become cancerous)
   - They can also find cases of DCIS and small cancers that would never cause symptoms or threaten a woman's life. This is called *over-diagnosis*. The treatment of over-diagnosed cancers and over-diagnosed cases of DCIS is not needed and results in *over-treatment*. Because doctors can't easily distinguish between cancers and cases of DCIS that need to be treated from those that do not, they are all treated
5. *Finding breast cancer early may not reduce a woman's chance of dying from the disease*

- Even though mammograms can detect cancerous tumors that can't be felt, treating a small tumor does not always mean that the woman will not die from the cancer. A fast-growing cancer may have already spread to other parts of the body before it is detected
- Finding breast cancer early may not help prolong the life of a woman who is suffering from other, more life-threatening health conditions

Colon Cancer

Colorectal cancer is a term used for a cancer that starts in the colon or the rectum. The colon begins in the right lower abdomen, near the appendix. It travels up the right side (ascending colon), crosses over the upper abdomen near the rib cage (transverse colon), and comes down the left side (descending colon). The last swing is called the *sigmoid colon*, which ends with the rectum and anus. The colon, also known as the *large intestine*, stores waste (e.g., poop, stool, BM), absorbs water (maintaining the body's water balance), absorbs some vitamins, and saves nutrients broken down by good intestinal bacteria.

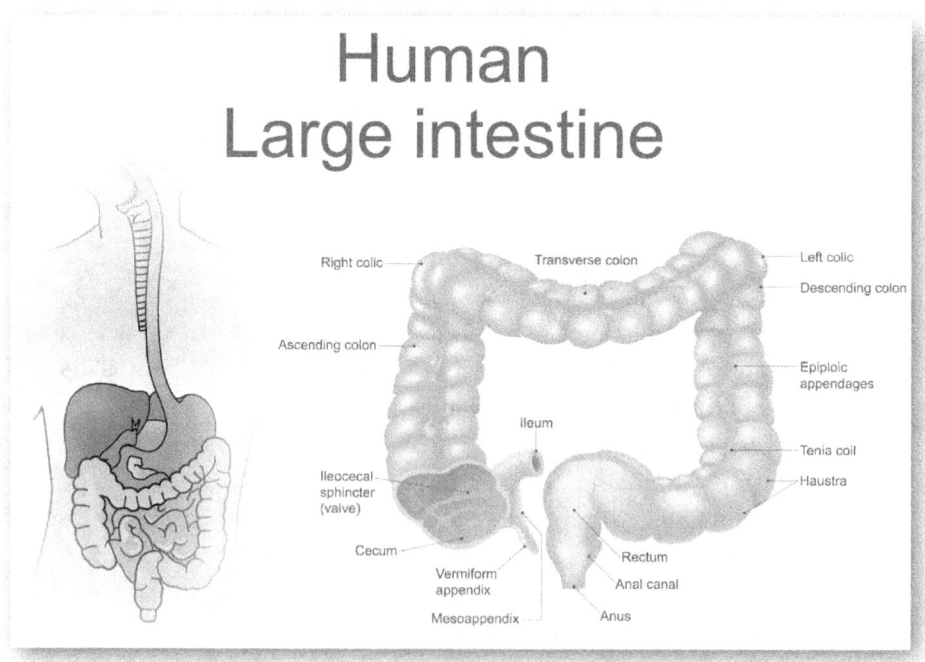

Most colorectal cancers develop slowly over several years, and commonly begin as a polyp. The *polyp*, an abnormal growth of the cells lining the colon, may be flush with the lining (like a mole or wart) or raised-up (like a balloon on a string). Some polyps can change into cancer, but not all do. If the cancer forms in a polyp, it can eventually begin to grow into the wall of the colon or rectum and spread to other parts of the body. The spreading of a cancer is called *metastasis*.

Colorectal cancer may cause one, or more, or none of these symptoms:

- A change in bowel habits, such as diarrhea, constipation, or narrowing of the stool, that lasts for more than a few days
- A feeling that you need to have a bowel movement that is not relieved by doing so
- Bleeding from the rectum
- Blood in the stool, which may cause the stool to look dark or black. (New blood is bright red, whereas old blood, from higher up in the intestinal tract, can look dark red or black)
- Cramping or abdominal (belly, stomach) pain
- Weakness and fatigue
- Unintended weight loss
- No symptoms at all

Because the symptoms of colon cancer can be very subtle or even nonexistent, screening is the best method of detection, and is recommended.

There are several ways to test for colon cancer. The first step, though, is to have a discussion with provider about your personal health history, risk factors, symptoms, and family history. Your provider will then guide you as to which testing methods are right for you.

When the time for the testing arrives, you may undergo one of two procedures, a *colonoscopy* or a *sigmoidoscopy* (detailed discussions of each follow). Because some foods or drugs can affect the test results, your provider may advise you to avoid the following in the days prior to these procedures:

- *Nonsteroidal anti-inflammatory drugs (NSAIDs)*: This includes ibuprofen (*Advil^R, Motrin^R*), naproxen (naprosyn, *Aleve^R*), or aspirin for seven days before testing. These medications have blood-thinning properties. If, during the procedure, a polyp needs to be removed, bleeding will be less likely to occur if these medications are stopped beforehand. NSAIDs can also cause bleeding due to irritation of the stomach or intestines. Small amounts of blood - blood that can't be seen unless a microscope is used - can cause a positive test when checking for blood in the stool (a sign of colon cancer) when there is actually no cancer present

- *Blood thinners*: for the reasons stated above
- *Vitamin C*: Refrain from taking more than 250 mg of Vitamin C daily from either supplements or citrus fruits and juices for three days before testing. Chemicals are used to check a stool sample for blood. Vitamin C can make the test negative, even when blood is present
- *Red meats (beef, lamb, or liver)*: Avoid eating these meats for three days before testing. Parts of blood in the meat may cause a positive test result when checking for blood in the stool, when in reality, you are not bleeding

Colon Cancer Screening Methods
Colonoscopy

A colonoscopy is a screening exam to look for colon cancer. During a colonoscopy, the provider is able to see inside your entire colon by using a *colonoscope* - a thin (it's about the thickness of a man's finger), flexible, hollow, lighted tube that has a tiny video camera on the end. The colonoscope is gently eased through the anus and inside the colon. From there it is able to send pictures to a computer screen. During this time, small amounts of air are puffed into the colon to keep it open, which helps the provider to see the entire colon clearly. While the procedure is being done, you are usually given medication through an IV in your arm to help you relax and sleep. The exam itself only takes about thirty minutes, although you will spend a significant amount of time prepping for the procedure (more on this to follow).

A colonoscopy is done by a *Gastroenterologist*, a specialist of the stomach and digestive system. A referral to the Gastroenterologist is typically made by your PCP for a "Screening Colonoscopy," and the procedure is covered under most health insurance plans as "Preventive Health." An office visit with the Gastroenterologist may or may not be done prior to the procedure.

Be sure the ordering provider and Gastroenterologist know about any medicines you are taking, as they may need to be changed before the test. If you normally take prescription medicines in the mornings, talk in advance with the providers, nurse, or receptionist about how to manage them for the day of the procedure.

When scheduling the procedure, have the name of the referring provider, your insurance card, and your pharmacy phone number available. A prescription for a laxative to clean out your colon will need to be filled.

Because you will not be allowed to eat before your colonoscopy, consider what time will work best for you and your health. (Most colonoscopies are scheduled in the morning hours.) Also, because a sedative is used to help you to relax and sleep during the procedure, you will need to arrange for someone you know to take you home after the test (not a cab or rideshare driver, as you may not be able to navigate stairs without assistance). Choose someone you trust, as the sedative may affect your memory.

The receptionist may give you an instruction sheet about the procedure if you schedule at the Gastroenterologist's office. If, after reading these instructions, you find you are not sure about *any* of the instructions, call the office and go over them step by step with the nurse or office assistant.

The day before your colonoscopy, you will begin a clear liquid diet, along with the prescription laxative, to clean out the colon. This prescription will be called into your neighborhood pharmacy by the Gastroenterologist's office (or if you receive a paper prescription, you will need to get it filled). *It is important to follow your instructions about the procedure prep very carefully.*

Avoid red and purple food colorings in all liquids, as these can be mistaken for blood in the colon. Permissible clear liquids typically include:

- Water, apple, or white grape juice, and any gelatin *except red or purple* for at least a day before the exam
- Clear broth, ginger ale, and usually most soft drinks or sports drinks *unless they have red or purple food colorings*
- Plain tea or coffee with sugar is usually okay, but no milk or creamer is allowed

As soon as you start taking the laxative, stay close to a bathroom. It is a good bet you will be most comfortable at home, in your own bathroom.

If the laxative is still working the morning of the colonoscopy, don't hesitate to ask where the bathroom is when you get to the facility. By the time you get there, all your bowel movements should be clear, like water. If you are not cleaned out well (if there is poop still left in your colon), the Gastroenterologist will not be able to get a good look around and may miss something important. They may even cancel the procedure because you are not cleaned out well enough. So it is extremely essential to take your laxatives and follow your diet as prescribed.

The Colonoscopy: Procedure

Once you arrive and have checked in, you will be taken back to the holding area and asked to take your clothes off and put on a gown. An IV will be started in your arm, and a small bag of hydrating fluid will be started. The Anesthesiologist (who will be giving you the sedative) may visit with you at this time You then will be wheeled into the procedure room and transferred onto a table. You may be asked to lie on your left side, with your knees flexed near your chest (laying on your left side allows easier access to the lower portion of the large intestine).

Just prior to the colonoscopy, the Anesthesiologist will give you a sedative through your IV. Shortly thereafter, you will fall asleep. For most people, this medicine causes them to be unaware of what is going on and unable to remember the procedure and any conversation afterward.

Your blood pressure, heart rate, breathing rate, and oxygen level will be monitored both during and after the test.

The colonoscopy usually takes about thirty minutes, but it may take longer if a polyp(s) is found and removed. If the Gastroenterologist sees a larger polyp, a tumor, or anything else abnormal, a *biopsy* may be done. For this procedure, a small piece of tissue is taken out through the colonoscope. The tissue is then looked at under a microscope by a Pathologist to determine if it is:

- Pre-cancerous (*adenoma*)
- Cancer
- Benign (not cancerous)
- A result of inflammation. The area may have increased redness and/or swelling as a result of irritation, infection, or other colon illness

When the procedure is completed, you will be taken back to the holding area. Due to the effects of the anesthesia, you will wake up after the test is over, but you might not be fully awake and cognizant until later in the day. Once you are awake enough to leave the facility, you will receive assistance with getting dressed (if needed), and discharged to your driver.

The results of the colonoscopy may be given to you while you are waiting to be discharged, or you may be asked to make a follow-up office appointment to review the colonoscopy findings. If the Gastroenterologist wishes to review the results with you while you are at the facility, it is important your driver be present to hear, as you may end up with no memory of what was said due to the medication given to you during the procedure. A discharge instruction sheet will also be sent home with you.

While it may be tempting not to schedule a recommended follow-up appointment, it is important to meet with the Gastroenterologist to review the results of your procedure. At this time, recommendations for future testing will be given, and any questions you have will be answered.

Sigmoidoscopy

During a sigmoidoscopy, a specially trained provider (physician, nurse practitioner, or physician's assistant) closely looks at *only* the lower part of the colon and the rectum through a scope similar to a colonoscope, but shorter, as it was not designed to go up as far. Because the scope is only about two feet long, the provider is able to see the entire rectum but only less than half of the colon.

Prior to the test, you must complete a bowel preparation by taking a prescribed laxative and/or an enema. A sigmoidoscopy usually takes ten to twenty minutes. Most people do not need to be sedated for this test, but this may be an option you can discuss with your provider. If a small polyp is found during the test, the provider may remove it with a small instrument passed through the scope. The polyp will be sent to a lab to be looked at by a Pathologist. If a pre-cancerous polyp (an *adenoma*) or colorectal cancer is found during the test, you will need to have a colonoscopy later to look for polyps or cancer in the rest of the colon.

Guidelines for Colon Cancer Screening for Men and Women of Average Risk

There are two main schools of thought for guideline recommendations for colon cancer screening.

1. American Cancer Society (ACS):
   www.cancer.org/cancer/colonandrectumcancer/moreinformation/
   colonandrectumcancerearlydetection/colorectal-cancer-early-detection-
   acs-recommendations

According to the American Cancer Society, both men and women at *average risk* for developing colorectal cancer should use *one* of the screening tests below beginning at age fifty. *Author's Note:* It is important you discuss with your PCP what your unique individual risk is. The ACS recommendations are as follows:

a. Colonoscopy: Every ten years

b. *OR* Sigmoidoscopy: Every five years (if results are abnormal, a colonoscopy will be recommended)

c. *OR* Double-contrast Barium Enema: Every five years

With this screening method, barium liquid is passed through the anus, and into the rectum and colon. An x-ray is taken, and if something abnormal is found, a colonoscopy will be recommended. A colon cleansing is required

d. *OR* CT Colonography (virtual colonoscopy): Every five years

A colon cleansing, similar to the colonoscopy will be required. With this method, you may be asked to drink a contrast solution before actually taking the test to help "tag" any remaining stool in your colon or rectum. The table you are laying on then slides into a CT scanner, and you will be asked to hold your breath while the scan takes place.

The CT scanner takes many pictures as it rotates around you while you are on the table. During the procedure, a small, flexible tube is inserted into your rectum, and air is pumped through the tube into the colon to provide better images. It is likely there will be two scans: one while you are laying on your back, and the other while you are laying on your stomach.

A computer then combines the pictures into images and creates slices of the part of your body being studied. If something abnormal is found, a colonoscopy will be recommended.

OR: (If any of the following tests results are abnormal, further testing will be recommended, since these tests are *mainly for cancer, not polyps.*)

e. Guaiac-based Fecal Occult Blood Test (gFOBT): Every year

This test checks for blood in the stool that can't be seen without using a microscope (blood can be an early sign of colon cancer). Your provider or the kit you receive will give you detailed instructions on how to collect the specimen.

To do this test, first have all of the supplies ready and in one place. These will include three test cards or slides and a brush or a wooden applicator. A toilet "hat" (an up-side-down top hat) may be provided to catch the stool, and there may be a mailing envelope included. If there is no envelope, a re-sealable bag can be used for transport. If possible, it is best to write your name and date on the cards before the stool sample is placed.

You collect the sample from your bowel movement (e.g., poop, stool). To place the toilet hat, lift the toilet lid and place the hat in up-side-down so it rests on the toilet bowl rim. Then lower the lid. If a toilet hat is not pro-vided, a sheet of plastic wrap or paper loosely draped across the toilet bowl can catch the stool, or you can use a dry, disposable container. Do not let the stool specimen mix with urine.

Use the wooden applicator or brush to smear a thin film of the stool sample onto one of the slots in the test card or slide. Next, collect a specimen from a different area of the same stool and smear a thin film of the sample onto the other slot in the test card or slide. There will only be two slots or places to smear the stool sample. After you obtain the samples, you can flush the remaining stool down the toilet.

Close the card, making sure your name and date are on the test kit cards. Store the cards overnight in a paper envelope to allow it time to dry. Repeat the test on your next two bowel movements, *each on a different day*, for a total of three stool samples. Place the test kit in the mailing pouch provided and return as instructed as soon as possible, but within 14 days of taking the first sample.

f.   Fecal immunochemical test (FIT): Every year

This test also checks for blood in the stool. The kit is obtained from your provider. It will give detailed instructions on how to collect the stool speci-men. Always follow the instructions on your kit.

Lift the toilet seat and position the sample collection paper across the rim of the toilet bowl. Secure the adhesive tabs to the sides of the toilet rim and lower the seat lid. Have a bowel movement onto the col-lection paper. Unscrew the cap from the sample collection tube. Poke the applicator into the stool at several sites. Screw the applicator back into the tube and secure tightly. Fill out the personal information on the attached label of the tube. Complete the address return label. Insert the sample collection tube into the specimen pouch and seal. Insert the sealed specimen pouch into the return envelope and seal. Return the sample packet immediately, as directed.

A similar type of test is available for over-the-counter use. Read all the instructions thoroughly and follow them exactly. Consult your provider if you have any questions or concerns.

g. Stool DNA test (sDNA): Every three years

A Stool DNA test looks for certain abnormal sections of DNA caused by cancer cells. Cells from colon and rectum cancers or polyps with these changes are often shed into the stool. *Cologuard*™ is able to check for these DNA changes and blood in the stool. After your provider has submitted the order, you will receive a kit in the mail to collect the stool samples. No special diet or bowel preparation (no laxatives or enemas) are required for a stool DNA test. The kit will contain a sample container, a bracket for holding the container in the toilet, a bottle of liquid preservative, a tube, labels, and a shipping box. The kit contains detailed instructions on how to collect the samples.

Place the bracket under the toilet seat and then put the toilet seat down. Remove the lid from the sample container (don't throw the lid away) and place it in the bracket. Sit on the toilet and try to have a bowel movement into the container. Try to keep urine from going in the container. When the bowel movement is complete, stand up and remove the container from the toilet and discard the bracket. Do not put toilet paper in the container.

Remove the cap from the tube that was included in the kit and pull the probe (like a stick) from the tube. Scrape the stool with the probe so that stool gets on the end. Put the probe back in the tube and screw the cap shut for Sample #1. Open the bottle of liquid preservative and pour all of the liquid over the stool in the container for Sample #2. Put the lid back on the sample container and screw it down tight. Label the samples and ship them according to the instructions in the kit. The samples should be sent within a day of collection.

2. U.S. Preventive Services Task Force (USPSTF):
www.uspreventiveservicestaskforce.org/Page/Document/ UpdateSummaryFinal/colorectal-cancer-screening2?ds=1&s=colon%20 cancer%20screening

a. Adults ages 50-75 years: Recommended screening starts at age 50 and continues to age 75. Encouragement is given to review the risk and benefits of the different testing methods with your provider

b. Adults ages 76-85 years: The decision to screen for colorectal cancer in adults aged 76 to 85 years should be an individual one, taking into account the patient's overall health and prior screening history

Tests that find *both cancer and polyps*:

- Flexible Sigmoidoscopy: Every five years
- Colonoscopy: Every ten years
- Double-contrast Barium Enema: Every five years
- CT Colonography (virtual colonoscopy): Every five years

Tests that mainly find cancer (*and not polyps*)

- Guaiac-based fecal occult blood test (gFOBT): Every year
- Fecal immunochemical test (FIT): Every year
- Stool DNA test (sDNA): Every three years

Cervical Cancer

Found only in females, the cervix is the bottom end part of the uterus (the womb; where a baby grows during pregnancy). It connects the uterus and the vagina (birth canal).

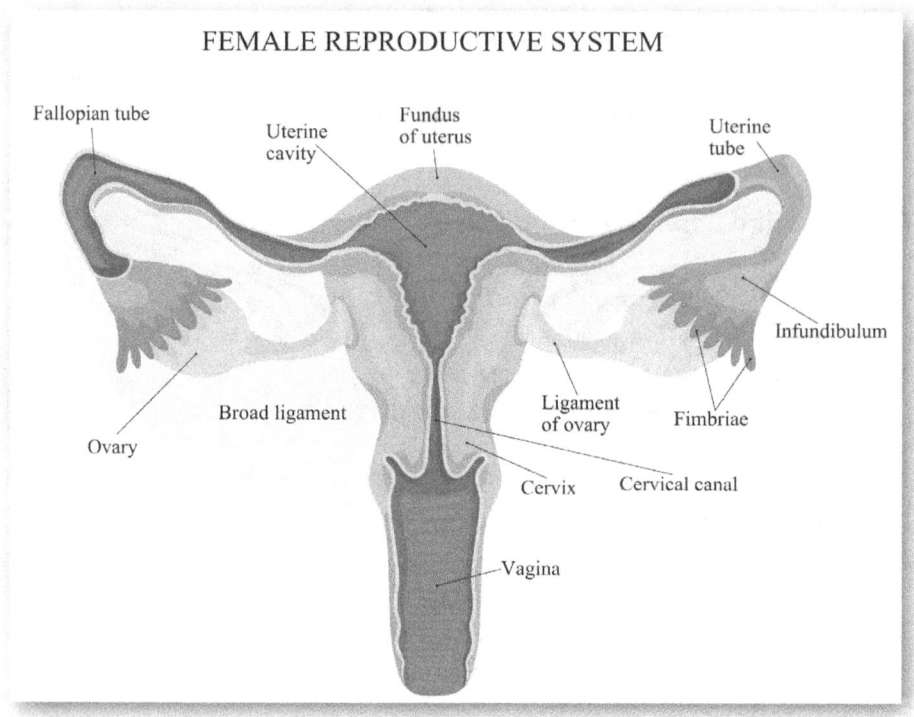

FEMALE REPRODUCTIVE SYSTEM

Fallopian tube

Uterine cavity

Fundus of uterus

Uterine tube

Infundibulum

Broad ligament

Ligament of ovary

Fimbriae

Ovary

Cervix

Cervical canal

Vagina

Most cases of *cervical* (cervix) cancer are caused by a virus called Human Papillomavirus (HPV). Of the 150 types of HPV, there are over forty types that are sexually transmitted and are considered a sexually transmitted disease (STD; sexually transmitted infection - STI). Each HPV *"type"* is given a number. It is possible to have more than one type of HPV.

Sexually transmitted HPV falls into two categories:

1. *Low-risk for cancer.* These types can cause genital warts in males and females, and are low-risk for causing cancer. The types responsible for most cases of genital warts are numbers 6 and 11.

2. *High-risk for cancer.* These types are responsible for causing genital cancer in both women (e.g., cervix, vagina) and in men (e.g., penis, anus). They are also responsible for causing cancer in the head and neck region (e.g., tongue, tonsils, and throat). The types responsible for most cases of cancer are numbers 16 and 18.

HPV is passed on with genital contact through vaginal or anal sex, oral sex, and genital-to-genital contact. A difficult part about having HPV is that you can pass it on to a sexual partner when you are having no symptoms and may not even know your are infected!

There are only two ways to know if someone has HPV. The first is that there are warts in the genital area (low-risk HPV). The second is by looking at a piece of tissue or a cell sample, obtained through a biopsy or Pap test.

When you have a Pap test (Pap smear), a *speculum* (this instrument looks very much like a duck's bill) is passed into your vagina until it reaches the cervix. At that point it is opened up (much like a duck opens its bill) so all of the cervix can be seen. The provider then obtains a sample of cells from the cervix by using a small brush or broom, and places them on a slide or in a special liquid. This sample is sent to the lab and viewed under a microscope.

If the cells are abnormal-appearing, an additional test (the HPV test) may be done to see if the cells have been affected by high-risk HPV. The Pap test and the HPV test are two different tests, but the same sample of cells can be used for both of them. If high-risk HPV is found, it may be recommended you have a *colposcopy* (biopsy) of the cervix. The Pathologist, who looks at the biopsy cells under the microscope, will be able to determine how damaged the cells are, and if cancer is present.

(*Author's Note:* If you are a female twenty-one years or older and have *never* had sexual intercourse [penis – vaginal penetration], talk with your provider about when you should start having Pap tests. Because the majority of cervical cancers are caused by high-risk HPV - a sexually transmitted disease - your risk for cervical cancer is extremely low. Likewise, if you and your male sexual partner were both virgins when you started having sexual intercourse and have only had sex with each other, your risk for having high-risk HPV is also low.)

Scheduling a Pap Test

When scheduling for a Pap test, there are several things you can do to make the test as accurate as possible:

- Try not to schedule an appointment during your menstrual period. The best time is at least five days after your period stops
- Don't use tampons, birth-control foams or jellies, other vaginal creams, mois-turizers, lubricants, or vaginal medicines for two to three days before the test.

(*Author's note:* Tampons should *never* be worn twenty-four hours a day, even if they are regularly changed. This can lead to a serious infection called *Toxic Shock Syndrome.* It is recommended that only pads be worn at some point in time, such as when asleep)

- Don't douche for two to three days before the test (In general, douching is never recommended)
- Don't have sexual intercourse for two days before the test
- If you are having any unusual vaginal drainage or odor, have this checked and treated before having your Pap test. This type of problem can affect the results

Paying for a Well-Woman Appointment and Pap Test

A well-woman exam, which includes a review of your sexual and menstrual history, breast exam and/or education, STD screening, and Pap test screening, is considered "Preventive Health" and will be covered by most insurance plans.

For those without insurance, a Pap test and STD screening may be obtained at privately or federally-funded health centers at a reduced fee, such as at your local Health Department or at Planned Parenthood. The Centers for Disease Control (CDC) also sponsors the National Breast and Cervical Cancer Early Detection Program (NBCCEDP), which provides access to breast and cervical cancer screening services to underserved women in all fifty states, the District of Columbia, five U.S. territories, and eleven tribes. This service supports programs that offer pelvic exams, Pap tests, and HPV screening. You may be eligible for free or low-cost screenings if you meet the following qualifications:

- Age 21–64
- Have no insurance, or the insurance does not cover screening exams
- Your yearly income is at or below 250 percent of the federal poverty level

Information about the NBCCEDP can be obtained by calling the CDC at 800-232-4636 or at their website: www.cdc.gov/cancer/nbccedp/about.htm.

HPV Vaccines

There is a vaccine available that prevents disease *and cancer* caused by the most common types of HPV. Because it falls under "Preventive Health", it may be covered by your health insurance plan. If you do not have health insurance, discuss with your PCP about places that offer the vaccine at a reduced fee. (Remember, HPV types 16 and 18 are high-risk for cancer, while types 6 and 11 are low-risk for cancer but can cause genital warts.)

a. *Gardasil 9* (protects against seven high-risk HPV types - 16, 18, 31, 33, 45, 52, and 58 and two low-risk types – 6 and 11)
Females and males: ages 9–26
www.cdc.gov/vaccines/hcp/vis/vis-statements/hpv-gardasil-9.html
(*Author's Notes:* Because women over the age of twenty-six were not included in the initial *Gardasil* studies, the FDA could not approve the vaccine for this age group. Since that time, studies have been conducted in women between the ages of twenty-seven and forty-five. Because the findings showed that the risk of infection and disease from HPV in this age group to be low, and that the vaccine didn't seem to benefit many women, the FDA concluded that the vaccine didn't help enough women to justify giving it to all women up to the age of forty-five.)

Pap Test Guidelines for Women of Average Risk

The cervical cancer screening guidelines are for women who are at *average* risk for cervical cancer and do not have any specific symptoms. This includes all women who are or ever have been sexually active (penis – vaginal penetration), even if they have had only one male partner and that male partner has had previous sex partners. There are two sets of recommendations. (*Author's Note:* Women who have had abnormal Pap smears and/or are positive for high-risk HPV may need to follow a different testing schedule. They should follow the recommendation of their provider.)

1. U. S. Preventive Services Task Force (USPSTF)
www.uspreventiveservicestaskforce.org/Page/Topic/recommendation-summary/cervical-cancer-screening?ds=1&s=cervical%20cancer
a. Women younger than 21: Recommends against screening for cervical cancer, as in 90 percent of cases of women this age, the body's immune system naturally clears the virus within two years
b. Women ages 21-65: Pap test every three years, *OR:*
▪ Women under 30: Recommends against routine screening for cervical cancer with just HPV testing alone, or in combination with a

Pap smear. (In other words, recommends just a Pap test every three years)

- Women ages 30-65 years who want to lengthen the screening interval: Screen with a combination of a Pap test and HPV testing every five years

c. Women 65 years and older: Recommends against screening for cervical cancer in women older than age sixty-five who have had adequate prior screening and are not otherwise at high-risk for cervical cancer

d. Women who have had a hysterectomy (removal of the uterus): Recommends against screening for cervical cancer in women who have had a hysterectomy with removal of the cervix and who do not have a history of a high-grade pre-cancerous lesion or cervical cancer

2. American Cancer Society
www.cancer.org/healthy/findcancerearly/cancerscreeningguidelines/chronological-history-of-acs-recommendations

a. Women ages 21-29: Pap every three years

b. Women ages 30-65: Pap test plus HPV test every five years. OR, screen with a Pap test alone every three years

c. Women over age 65: Stop screening unless the patient has had a serious cervical pre-cancer or cancer in the last twenty years

Prostate Cancer

Found only in males, the prostate gland is located below the *bladder* (the organ that holds urine) and in front of the rectum. The size of the prostate gland changes with age. In younger men, it is about the size of a walnut, but it can grow much larger in older men.

The prostate's job is to make some of the fluid that protects and nourishes the sperm cells in semen, and makes the semen more liquid. The *urethra*, the tube that carries urine and semen out of the body through the penis, goes through the center of the prostate gland.

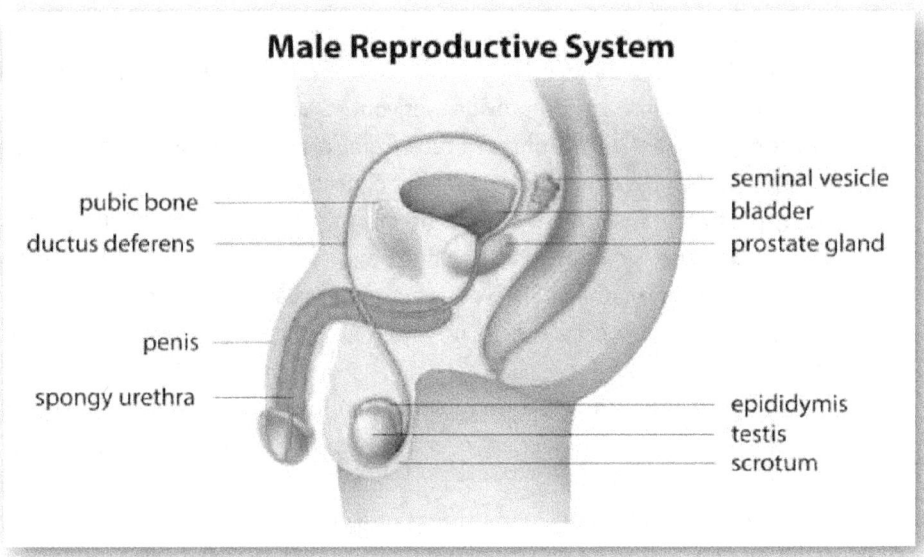

Nearly all prostate cancers develop from the *gland cells*, which are the cells that make the prostate fluid that is added to the semen. Some prostate cancers can grow and spread quickly, but most grow slowly.

Prostate Cancer Screening Methods

Screening for prostate cancer can be done two ways, which are usually used together.

a. PSA: Prostate-Specific Antigen blood test

    PSA, a substance made by cells in the prostate gland, is mostly found in semen, but a small amount is also found in the blood.

    The PSA blood test measures the amount of PSA in a man's blood. As the PSA level in the blood goes up, the chance of having prostate cancer also goes up. Most healthy men have levels under 4 (ng/mL). When prostate cancer develops, the PSA level usually goes above 4 (although there is still a chance for men to have prostate cancer with a level below 4)

b. Digital Rectal Exam (DRE)

    For a DRE, your provider inserts a gloved, lubricated finger into your rectum to feel for any bumps or hard areas on the prostate gland that might be cancer.

With the DRE, the prostate may feel very normal to your provider, but the results of your PSA blood test may be elevated. On the other hand, your prostate may feel lumpy and hard to your provider, yet your PSA blood test may be normal.

If the result of either one of these tests is abnormal, a biopsy of the prostate tissue may be recommended to look for cancer.

Early prostate cancer usually causes no symptoms. But more advanced prostate cancer can sometimes cause symptoms, such as:

- Problems urinating: a slow or weak urine stream, or the need to urinate more often, especially at night
- Blood in the urine
- Trouble getting an erection (erectile dysfunction)
- Pain in the hips, back, chest, or other areas from prostate cancer that has spread to the bones
- Weakness or numbness in the legs or feet
- Loss of bladder or bowel control (leaking urine or stool without intending to)

Prostate Cancer Screening Guidelines

1. U. S. Preventive Services Task Force (USPSTF)
   www.uspreventiveservicestaskforce.org/Page/Topic/recommendation-summary/prostate-cancer-screening?ds=1&s=prostate%20cancer
   - Recommends against prostate-specific antigen (PSA)-based screening for prostate cancer (blood test)

   (Author's note: As of this writing, this topic is in the process of being updated by the USPSTF)

2. American Cancer Society
   www.cancer.org/cancer/prostatecancer/moreinformation/prostatecancer earlydetection/prostate-cancer-early-detection-acs-recommendations
   Men should have a chance to make an informed decision with their healthcare provider about whether to be screened for prostate cancer. The decision should be made after getting information about the uncertainties, risks, and potential benefits of prostate cancer screening.

A. *Guidelines for Prostate Cancer Screening for Men Ages 50 and Older Who Are of Average Risk*

1. Providers should begin discussion with men aged fifty who have at least a ten-year life expectancy
2. If the PSA is 2.5 ng/ml or greater, testing should be repeated yearly
3. Men with a PSA of less than 2.5 ng/ml may be tested every other year

B. *Guidelines for Prostate Cancer Screening for Men Ages 45 years and Older Who Are High-risk*

1. High-risk men:
   - African-American men
   - Men with a strong family history of prostate cancer (e.g., two or more affected first-degree relatives - father, brother, son)
   - Men with a strong family history of one or more first-degree relatives (father, brother, son) who were diagnosed younger than 65 years of age
2. If the PSA is 2.5 ng/ml or greater, testing should be repeated yearly
3. Men with a PSA of less than 2.5 ng/ml may be tested every other year

The Risks and Benefits of Prostate Cancer Screening
Benefits:

- For men with an aggressive prostate cancer, treatment can be started earlier in the course of the disease, possibly before it has spread
- The five-year survival for men with prostate cancer confined to the prostate is nearly 100 percent. This drops to 30 percent for men whose cancer has spread to other areas of the body
- The screening tests are not perfect but are easy to perform and have fair accuracy

Risks:

- Screening for prostate cancer may not improve your health or help you to live longer if the prostate cancer has already spread to other places in your body
- Some prostate cancers never have symptoms or are life-threatening. It is un-known if screening for these cancers help you to live longer, than if left unde-tected with no treatment given
- Screening detects many prostate cancers which are unlikely to cause death or disability. It is not clear that all prostate cancers must be treated
- False-negatives results (occurs when no abnormality is identified even though prostate cancer is present) and false-positive results (occurs when an abnormality is identified even though there is no cancer present) can occur

After the discussion about screening with their provider, those men who want to be screened should be tested with the prostate-specific antigen (PSA) blood test. The digital rectal exam (DRE) may also be done as a part of screening.

CHAPTER 8

Legal Documents, In Case Of...

(Is all this really necessary?)

A t some point in time - a time that many of us all-too-easily-and-uncomfortably push aside until "later" - we must consider having a plan in place in the event that we become:

- *Terminally ill* (death is just around the corner)
- *Permanently unconscious or in a vegetative state* (permanently lose the ability to interact with our environment and communicate with our loved ones)
- Unable to make your own healthcare decisions because of mental or physical incapacitation

With such a tough and heartbreaking possibility in mind, I am going to briefly review the legal documents that allow others to make decisions for you when you are unable to do so.

End-of-Life Care Decisions
(The care you wish to receive should you become terminally ill, permanently unconscious, or unable to make your own healthcare decisions)

A difficult yet important legal arrangement to consider is the making of End-of-Life Care decisions. All of the states have made it possible for their residents to give detailed instructions regarding the kind of care they would like to receive should they become terminally ill, permanently unconscious, or unable to make their own healthcare decisions. Depending on which state they live in, this may take the form of a healthcare proxy/healthcare power of attorney/durable power of attorney for healthcare, a medical/advance directive, a living will, or a combination thereof.

Appointing an Agent

Regardless of what type of power of attorney you use, it is important to think carefully about who you will chose to be your *agent* - the one who agrees and is authorized to act on your behalf. Your agent will have a lot of control over your finances and/or healthcare, so it is crucial that you trust them completely. Know too that all powers of attorney that you grant come to an end at your death. In other words, your agent will have no power to make any decisions after you die.

Since your agent will have the authority to make decisions in the event you are unable to make such decisions for yourself, the agent should be a family member or friend that you trust to follow your instructions. Before executing a healthcare proxy/ healthcare power of attorney, you should talk to the person whom you want to name as the agent about your wishes concerning medical and financial decisions, especially life-sustaining treatment.

Power Of Attorney

*(You, the patient, give the agent **financial** control)*

A *"power of attorney"* is a legal document in which you (the *"principal"*) appoint someone else - the *"agent"* or *"attorney-in-fact"* - to act for you in regards to your financial and business affairs.

This agent can do any business or monetary-related act you need them to do in the event you become incapacitated or can't act on your own behalf. Otherwise, if you don't have a power of attorney and become suddenly incapacitated, your family may have to go through an expensive and time-consuming court action to appoint a guardian or conservator to make financial and business decisions for you.

- A **general** or **conventional** power of attorney is comprehensive in scope: It gives your agent all the powers and rights that you have yourself. For example, a general power of attorney may give your agent the right to sign documents, pay bills, and conduct financial transactions on your behalf. (*Author's Note: You also can use a general power of attorney even if you are not incapacitated, but still need someone to help with financial matters.*)

A general power of attorney *ends on your death or incapacitation*, unless canceled by you when you are not incapacitated.

- A **durable** power of attorney can be general or limited in scope, but it remains in effect *after* you become incapacitated. A durable power of attorney will remain *in effect until your death*, unless canceled by you when not incapacitated.

- A **springing** power of attorney allows your agent to act for you if you become incapacitated. Unlike a durable power of attorney, it does not become effective *until* you are incapacitated.

  If you are using a springing power of attorney, it is very important that the document contain a very detailed description of what you view as incapacitated *and* a clear-cut statement declaring when the agent is to take over legal financial power.

- A **limited** power of attorney gives someone else the power to act on your behalf for a very limited purpose. For example, a limited power of attorney could give someone the right to sign a property deed for you on a day when you are out of town. It usually ends at a time specified in the document.

Healthcare Proxy; Healthcare Power of Attorney; Durable Power of Attorney for Healthcare

(*You, the patient, give the agent control of **health-related** decisions.*)

If you become incapacitated, it is important that someone have the legal authority to communicate your wishes concerning your *medical treatment*.

Similar to a power of attorney, a *healthcare proxy/healthcare power of attorney* allows you to appoint someone else to act as your agent, but for medical (as opposed to financial) decisions. The healthcare proxy/healthcare power of attorney is a document carried out by you (the *principal*, or the *patient*, who is competent), giving another person (the *agent*) the authority to make healthcare decisions for you if you are unable to communicate such decisions.

By executing a healthcare proxy/healthcare power of attorney, you are guaranteeing that your instructions and wishes – which you should have provided to your agent via a Medical or Advance Directive (see discussion that follows) - will be carried out by your designated agent. This is wise to do if you have a partner, spouse, children, or relatives who may feel differently about, or disagree with, your desired treatment.

In general, a healthcare proxy/healthcare power of attorney takes effect *only when you require medical treatment, and a physician determines that you are unable to communicate your wishes concerning treatment.* (*Author's Note:* How this works exactly can depend on the laws of the particular state and the terms of the healthcare proxy/ healthcare power of attorney itself.) If you later become able to express your own wishes, your provider(s) will listen to your wishes, and the healthcare proxy/healthcare power of attorney will no longer be in effect.

Medical Directive; Advance Directive

(*You, the patient, give the healthcare agent* **specific instructions** *on the type of healthcare you want to receive.*)

Accompanying a healthcare proxy/healthcare power of attorney should be a *Medical Directive,* also called an *Advance Directive.* This directive provides the agent with specific instructions as to *what type of medical care you would like.* It may be included in the healthcare proxy/healthcare power of attorney, or be a separate, standalone document.

This directive may contain directions to refuse, remove, or allow life support in the event you, the patient, are in a coma or a vegetative state. It also may list specific procedures and treatments you choose or decline, such IV fluids (fluid from a bag into the vein), a feeding tube in your stomach, life-saving medications, surgery, blood transfusions, and oxygen.

(*Author's Note:* Remember that a *general power of attorney,* which is intended for financial matters, will not grant any rights regarding your medical decisions. You need a healthcare proxy/healthcare power of attorney for that.)

Living Wills

(*You, the patient, request the* **withdrawal of life support** *in instances of terminal illness, coma, or vegetative state.*)

Living wills are documents that give detailed instructions regarding withdrawal of your life support treatment should you become terminally ill, are in a persistent vegetative state, or are unable to communicate your own decisions. The living will states under what conditions life-sustaining treatment should be terminated.

It is important to note there is a huge difference between a living will, which states under what conditions life-sustaining treatment should be terminated, and a *"Do Not Resuscitate" order (DNR)*. A DNR order says that if you are having a medical emergency, such as a heart attack or stroke, and your heart stops beating or you stop breathing, medical professionals are not to try to revive (resuscitate) you. This is very different from a living will, *which only goes into effect when you are already in a vegetative state.*

Like a healthcare proxy/healthcare power of attorney, a living will takes effect *when* you become incapacitated and are unable to make your own decisions. A living will is not set in stone; you can always revoke it at a later date if you wish to do so.

A living will, however, is not necessarily a substitute for a healthcare proxy/healthcare power of attorney or broader medical/advance directive. *It only addresses the withdrawal of life support in instances of terminal illness, coma or a vegetative state,* when you cannot purposely respond to any interaction, as with speaking or following commands.

While many pre-packaged, do-it-yourself power of attorney and healthcare proxy forms are available, it is a good idea to have an *Elder attorney*, who is a specialist in this field, draft the form specifically for you. There are many issues to consider, and one size does not fit all. Each state has different wording, notary, and witness requirements for living wills, so do-it-yourself forms and requirements vary from state to state.

To learn more, contact an Elder Law attorney. Or, many hospitals and nursing homes also provide forms, which you can complete with help from the facility's Social Services/Care Management department.

POLST: A New Approach

Although medical/advance directives and/or living wills provide general guidance on what type of care you would like, they are not consistently followed, in part because they don't give healthcare professionals explicit instructions for making critical decisions about your care. An alternative option has emerged in recent years and has been implemented or is being developed in many states. The name varies, depending on the state:

- Physician Orders for Life-Sustaining Treatment (POLST)
- Medical Orders for Life-Sustaining Treatment (MOLST)
- Clinician Orders for Life-Sustaining Treatment (COLST)
- Physician Orders for Scope of Treatment (POST)

POLST uses a standardized medical order form on which you indicate which types of life-sustaining treatment you want or don't want if seriously ill, or if your condition worsens. You or your healthcare proxy/healthcare power of attorney must sign it, *as well as a healthcare provider*.

Keep your POLST paperwork with your other end-of-life documents. Have them close by in the event of illness or emergency. *Author's Note:* POLST does not replace a Medical/Advanced Directive.

Wills

Another very important document to consider making is your will. While many people do not wish to think about their own death, it is something that will happen.

There is no better way to control who gets what after your death than a will. Planning in advance will save your family and loved ones time, money, and a great deal of stress.

Your *estate* consists of all your personal items, money, real estate, and/or intellectual properties, such as copyrights and trademarks. These possessions, which may or may not be of great value, can be passed on to the person(s) of your choosing. The *beneficiary* (or beneficiaries) is the person whom you designate to receive any or all of your property.

A *will* is a legal document in which you declare who will manage your estate after you die. This person, the *executor,* is the individual whom you name who will be responsible for fulfilling your wishes as outlined in the will.

Having a will also will allow you to declare who is to be the *guardian* of any minor children or dependents.

It is important to have a will, because if you die *without* a valid will:

- Your estate (possessions) will become *intestate*. This means your estate will be settled based on the laws of your state. (If you do have a will, it is called *testate*)
- The judge will appoint an *administrator* to serve as the executor. This designated administrator may be a stranger to you and your family, and they are bound by the letter of the probate laws of your state. (*Probate* is the legal process of transferring the property of a deceased person to the rightful heirs.) As such, this administrator may make decisions that wouldn't necessarily agree with your wishes or those of your heirs

If you die and *do* have a will, your will be reviewed by the probate court to ensure it complies with state law. The court can also supervise the actions of your appointed executor. Some states may allow for accelerated probate procedures, depending on the size of the estate. In order to avoid the probate process, you can set up a *trust*, name a *trustee* (the individual responsible for distributing your assets), and designate the beneficiaries of the property in your will. (All property must be re-titled in the name of the trust.)

There are types of property that are not generally covered by a will. These may include:

- property owned in survivorship with another person
- life insurance proceeds
- accounts payable on death
- insurance policies
- retirement accounts
- property you have transferred into a trust

If any of the types of property on the aforementioned list pertain to you, simply check to make sure a beneficiary of your choosing has been named to each account.

You do not require an attorney to prepare a will, as you can find forms for drafting a will online. Consulting with a *licensed attorney*, or more specifically, an *elder attorney* (a specialist in elder law), can provide you with legal peace-of-mind by guaranteeing all state and federal requirements have been met in your will. They can also assist with *estate planning*, the creation and collection of legal documents that clearly communicate your end-of-life wishes. With their help, you can be confident your wishes will be carried out before and after your passing.

Clarification Summary

- *Power of Attorney*: You give the agent *financial* control of your affairs
- *Healthcare Proxy; Healthcare Power of Attorney; Durable Power of Attorney for Healthcare*: You give the agent control of *health*-related decisions as they pertain to you
- *Medical Directive; Advance Directive*: You give the agent *specific instructions* on the *type of healthcare* you want to receive, such as a breathing tube, feeding tube, or dialysis; organ, tissue, or body donation

- *Living Will*: You request *the withdrawal of life support* in instances of terminal illness, coma, or a vegetative state, which only goes into effect *once you are already in a vegetative state*
- *Do Not Resuscitate Order*: *This prevents medical personnel from administering lifesaving methods*, such CPR (chest compressions) and intubation (breathing tube into the lungs), *in the event your heart stops beating or you stop breathing*

Over Time...

Once you have your desired healthcare documents drawn up, your agent should keep the original document. You should have a copy and your PCP should keep a copy with your medical records. Consider giving copies of them to a trusted friend and/or family member, clergy, and the hospital on admission. If possible, upload them into your Electronic and Personal Health Record. Also, keep your agent's name and contact information in your wallet in the event of an emergency.

If you wish to make any changes to your healthcare documents as time passes, know that the changes must be written down, signed, and dated. Then give copies of them to your family, agent, and provider, having them dispose of the old document.

If you are making substantial changes to one document in particular, ensure an entirely new document is drawn up, written, and witnessed.

It is important to know that state laws vary concerning end-of-life documentation. All fifty states allow you to express your wishes as to medical treatment, and to appoint someone to communicate those wishes should you be unable to do so. But, consider the following differences:

- The names of these documents may vary from state to state
- Some states require a standardized form, while others allow you to draft your own document
- An Advance/Medical Directive drafted in one state may not work in another state. If this applies to you, it is recommended you complete an Advance/Medical Directive in each state involved, according to each state's guidelines
- Emergency Medical Services (EMS) is the response team to a medical emergency. They can be summoned by dialing 911 and asking for an ambulance. If EMS is called for someone who has an Advance/Medical Directive, POLST,

and/or Do Not Resuscitate (DNR) order, have the paperwork available when the responders arrive. After assessing the patient, EMS may or may not be able to honor the patient's wishes. Their Advance/Medical Directive policy varies from state to state

- The National Hospice and Palliative Care Organization sponsor a website that allows you to view and download your state's Advance Directive requirements and documentation: www.caringinfo.org/i4a/pages/index. cfm?pageid=3289

CHAPTER 9

Healthcare Dos, Don'ts, and Lifesavers

(Patient-Tested Tips and Techniques)

This chapter contains a summary of keys points every patient should be aware of. Listing them as I have done will give you brief yet straight forward pieces of information that can improve your healthcare experience as a patient.

For reinforcement, I have intentionally pulled specific recommendations from the previous chapters, and added to them other insightful observations and helpful tips.

1. *Realize another's medical story is personal and unique to them, and may not be applicable to you – at all.* Your acquaintances will be more than happy to share their provider and health information with you, be it good or bad. Remember when talking to others about their healthcare that *everyone* has a story. Some are more willing than others to share it with you, whether you want to hear it or not. As you hear it, consider who is saying what, how they are saying it, and if the information seems reliable. It remains *your choice* whether to use that information and apply it to your own experience – or not. What happened to them may have absolutely no bearing on your own experience

2. *Be cautious of sites that "grade" providers.* This information can be very inconsistent. The fewer number of reviews, the less likely they are a true representation of the provider

3. Choosing to establish with a provider located near you will make it easier for you to make and keep appointments

4. Keep an updated health history with you at all times, in case of an emergency. This list should include diagnoses, medications (name of; what they're for; dose; taken how often; and who the prescriber is), surgeries, names of your providers, and medication allergies. Or, install a medical history app on your cell phone (see below)

5. *Take advantage of medical apps.* For example, there are apps to help you:
    - Remember to take your medication
    - Relax
    - Keep journals to track your migraines, menstrual periods, menopause symptoms, and/or sleep patterns
    - Allow you to manage and monitor pain
    - Lose weight
    - Record numbers, such as for high blood pressure and diabetes

    In addition: *Install a Medical History app on your phone.* It can be a life-saver! With this app, your medical information can be easily found on your phone - in case of a medical emergency. Emergency medical personnel can see your medical history on your phone, without the need of a passcode.

    Some phones and apps also offer you the option to designate a contact person - *ICE: In Case of Emergency* – whose name can be found without anyone using a passcode

6. *Please, please, please, tell the lab technician in advance if you are scheduled to have blood drawn and have been known to pass out during this procedure.* Lab technicians know this reaction can't be helped, and having you pass out on a table or in a reclining chair is far more manageable than having you pass out in an upright lab chair

7. *Following-up on medical test results.* When your provider orders a test of any kind, ask how you will be notified of the results, and in what time frame. Some providers will call with your results, others will send a letter. Many providers will only contact you with abnormal results. Or, you may receive the results through the EHR or PHR. Be conscious of whether you receive the news in the expected time frame. If you do not hear back and want to know what the results are, call or go to the office as many times as necessary to get the requested information

8. *Don't bring in copies of your old x-rays unless the provider specifically asks for them.* Choosing to bring in printed reports from the Radiologist may prove more helpful. Also, many times a provider can obtain necessary reports and actual x-rays from the Electronic Health Record

9. *If you encounter a somewhat brusque individual in the medical world, try not to let it hurt your feelings.* Not everyone in healthcare has a pleasant demeanor. Not everyone in any profession has a pleasant demeanor

10. *Waiting in healthcare is unavoidable, so come prepared.* Emergencies arise, and vast amounts of people need to be seen, both for well and sick visits. Bring materials to any visits that allow you (and any family members) to pass the time in an enjoyable fashion

11. *Never, ever be afraid to ask a question.* Truly, there are no stupid questions in healthcare. Know that you will not be the first, or the last, to ask the specific question that is on your mind

12. *Be cautious when surfing the web to find answers to your medical questions.* Finding what is true and accurate on the Internet can be a challenge. Don't believe everything you read, and don't let information you come upon turn you into an alarmist. Consult with your provider about your questions

13. *If your illness is controlled when taking medication, such as for high blood pressure or diabetes, don't stop taking the medication if your numbers become normal, unless instructed to do so by your provider.* Your numbers are normal because you *are* taking the medication

14. *Reply to healthcare surveys, detailing whether your experience was good or bad.* After any procedure (e.g., lab draw, mammogram, x-ray), office visit, or hospital stay, you may receive a survey in the mail or online. Survey responses allow the staff at the healthcare system to see what they are doing well, and what needs improvement. If you had a positive experience, return the survey with a positive response. If you did not have a positive experience, respond with the specific reasons why

15. *If you wish to acknowledge a particular caregiver or group, consider sending a card, flowers, or food (pre-packaged or delivered from a restaurant).* Many hospitals, clinics, and healthcare systems have policies that restrict their employees from accepting gifts, other than those of minimal value (e.g., floral arrangements, cards, and food). If you want to show your appreciation to a healthcare giver, but are unsure of the best way to do it,

contact the business's Human Resources department to help answer that question

16. *Expect from yourself what you expect from your provider.* Your primary care provider and support staff want you to be well, and stay well. Everything they do is to assist *you* in living a happy and healthy life. Bearing this in mind, it is important that you are a participant in your own healing. If you don't try - not taking your medications as prescribed; not following-up as scheduled; not doing procedures as ordered - how can you expect your provider to make things all better? You can't expect the provider to keep you well without your cooperation

17. *If something seems "off," be proactive, and double-check that what is going on is correct.* Every player in your healthcare team is working together to benefit you. Yet because this is not a perfect world, the communication between each player in healthcare may not always be consistent. Protect yourself by:
   - Asking questions
   - Keeping your medical paperwork organized
   - Following-up if you receive no response, or conflicting or confusing responses
   - Documenting conversations with dates, names, and times

   Being proactive will help lessen your stress in the territory of healthcare

18. *Involve at least one close family member or friend in your healthcare.* It is prudent to have somebody as a backup should you become incapacitated or forgetful – or just need somebody you can trust to bounce ideas off, or offer up their opinion

19. *Write down all the information that will be helpful in the event of your death and give it to someone you can trust or place it in a safety deposit box*, such as:
   - Location of your will, living will, trust papers, and other legal documents (*See Chapter 8 for a description of these*)
   - Banks with account numbers
   - Investment houses with account numbers
   - Life insurance policy
   - Safety deposit box key location, number on the box, and bank located in
   - Passwords: email, Facebook, online businesses, etc.
   - Credit and debit cards, and their respective account numbers
   - Loan payment information
   - Social security card or number

- Health insurance names and numbers
- Place of employment contact information
- Preference of funeral home, and any burial requests
- Immediate family members' contact information

20. *Know that providers order tests for three reasons*:
    a. To identify a problem or condition
    b. To monitor the problem or condition
    c. To rule out a problem or condition

    When your provider has a test done and the result is normal or negative, they can then eliminate a potential diagnosis. For example, if a patient is concerned about how well their thyroid is functioning, normal thyroid blood tests can eliminate this concern

21. *Money plays an important part in healthcare, so plan and research all your financial options accordingly.* There is little or no way around this reality. However, do plan to take advantage of any health fairs offered in your community. Many offer health screenings and fasting lab tests at a reduced fee. If a result is abnormal or you are unsure of what the result means, follow-up with your primary care provider

22. *Comparison-price-shop.* There are many ways you can end up saving money when it comes to your healthcare without jeopardizing quality of care:
    - Contact various diagnostic centers as to their prices for medical services and tests. Have the order in hand, so you can say *exactly* what tests have been ordered. Doing so can save money for both those with and without insurance
    - If you have an insurance plan, view the company's website, as it may provide options for price comparison

23. *Keep all medication, prescription and over-the-counter, out of the reach of children and all others who might be interested in trying it*

24. *Take a prefilled medication box with you on vacation.* It is very easy to get off schedule and forget to take your medication while away. By taking a pre-filled medication box, you will know by looking at it if you took your medication that day. It is recommended that you also take the container the medication comes in, as the label will include important prescription information, if needed. Use a medical app that helps you remember whether or not you took your medication. Always keep your medication with you when traveling in the event you are separated from your luggage

25. *If you are seeing multiple providers, consider separate binders for each provider to help organize names, specialties, appointments, instructions, medications, and billing*

26. *Consider price shopping for medications.* In some instances, the cash price (what you pay out-of-pocket) of the medication is less expensive than what your insurance company will charge. For those without insurance, call around to the different pharmacies to compare prices

27. *If, during your illness, you choose to take someone else's medication or a medication from another country, write down the name of that medication and bring it with you to your office visit, should you continue to not feel well.* While your provider may not be happy that you took it, it will be important for them to know what it was, when deciding your plan of care

28. *Confirm that every provider who performs a medical service is in your health insurance network.* This includes clinic settings, the Urgent Care, the Emergency Room, and *all* hospital providers

29. *If you have not been to your PCP within a certain amount of time (for example, three years), the clinic may no longer view you as an established patient when you call to schedule an appointment.* You may now be considered a new patient. And if your clinic is no longer accepting new patients, you may no longer be able to be seen there

30. *If you have insurance and need to have a procedure or surgery done, your provider may ask for part or all of your deductible in payment first.* This assures that the provider will be paid for their services

31. *Just because you have insurance, doesn't mean you have to use it.* When researching prices, you may find that the cash price (your out-of-pocket cost) is less than what your insurance will bill you. This is especially true for some medications and lab tests. While the amount paid may not be applied toward your deductible, this option may be financially beneficial for those unlikely to meet their deductible in an insurance calendar year

CHAPTER 10

Your Rights as a Patient
(*Who knew?*)

This chapter covers the *Patient's Bill of Rights*. The *Patient's Bill of Rights* was first created by the American Hospital Association (AHA) in 1973 and was later revised in 1992. *They were developed with the expectation that hospitals and healthcare institutions would support these rights in the interest of delivering effective patient care.*

Following the AHA's initiative, President Clinton created the U.S. Advisory Commission on Consumer Protection and Quality in the Healthcare Industry in 1998. The Commission's purpose was to advise the President on changes occurring in the healthcare system and recommend measures necessary to promote and assure healthcare quality and value, and protect consumers and workers in the healthcare system. Building off of the original Patient Bill of Rights, this commission was created to reach three major goals:

1. To help patients feel more confident in the U.S. healthcare system:
   - Assures that the healthcare system is fair, and that it works to meet the patients' needs
   - Gives patients a way to address any problems they may have
   - Encourages patients to take an active role in staying or getting healthy
2. To stress the importance of a strong relationship between patients and their healthcare providers
3. To stress the key role patients play in staying healthy by laying out rights and responsibilities for all patients and healthcare providers

There are eight key areas the Patient's Bill of Rights was designed to protect:

1. Information for patients: You have the right to accurate and easily understood information about your health plan, healthcare professionals, and healthcare facilities. So, for example, if you speak another language, have a physical or mental disability, or just don't understand something, help should be given so you can make informed healthcare decisions.

2. Choice of providers and plans: You have the right to choose healthcare providers who can give you high-quality healthcare when you need it. To ensure this choice, health plans should provide access to an adequate provider network, qualified Women's healthcare specialists, specialists, and transitional care.

3. Access to emergency services: If you have severe pain, an injury, or a sudden illness that causes you to believe that your health is in danger, you have the right to be screened and stabilized using emergency services. You should be able to use these services whenever and wherever you need them, without needing to wait for authorization and without any financial penalty.

4. Taking part in treatment decisions: You have the right to know your treatment options and take part in decisions about your care. Parents, guardians, family members, or others that you choose can speak for you if you cannot make your own decisions.

5. Respect and non-discrimination: You have a right to considerate, respectful care from your doctors, health plan representatives, and other healthcare providers that do not discriminate against you.

6. Confidentiality (privacy) of health information: You have the right to talk privately with healthcare providers and to have your healthcare information protected. You also have the right to read and copy your own medical record. You have the right to ask that your doctor change your record if it is not correct, relevant, or complete.

7. Complaints and appeals: You have the right to a fair, fast, and objective review of any complaint you have against your health plan, doctors, hospitals, or other healthcare personnel. This includes complaints about waiting times, operating hours, the actions of healthcare personnel, and the adequacy of healthcare facilities.

8. <u>Consumer responsibilities</u>: In a healthcare system that protects consumer or patients' rights, patients should expect to take on some responsibilities to get well and/or stay well (for instance, exercising and not using tobacco). Patients are expected to do things like treat healthcare workers and other patients with respect, try to pay their medical bills, and follow the rules and benefits of their health plan coverage. Having patients involved in their care increases the chance of the best possible outcomes and helps support a high quality, cost-conscious healthcare system.

On the following pages, you will find many examples of a Patient Bill's of Rights, each specifically designed to meet the needs of the parent organization, as was encouraged by the AHA in their original version.

American Hospital Association: The Patient Care Partnership (2003)

What to Expect During Your Hospital Stay:

1. <u>High quality hospital care</u>: Our first priority is to provide you the care you need, when you need it, with skill, compassion, and respect. Tell your caregivers if you have concerns about your care or if you have pain. You have the right to know the identity of doctors, nurses, and others involved in your care, and you have the right to know when they are students, Residents, or other trainees.

2. <u>A clean and safe environment</u>: Our hospital works hard to keep you safe. We use special policies and procedures to avoid mistakes in your care and keep you free from abuse or neglect. If anything unexpected and significant happens during your hospital stay, you will be told what happened and any resulting changes in your care will be discussed with you.

3. <u>Involvement in your care</u>: You and your doctor often make decisions about your care before you go to the hospital. Other times, especially in emergencies, those decisions are made during your hospital stay. When decision-making takes place, it should include:

   a. Discussing your medical condition and information about medically appropriate treatment choices. To make informed decisions with your doctor, you need to understand:

- The benefits and risks of each treatment
- Whether your treatment is experimental or part of a research study
- What you can reasonably expect from your treatment and any long-term effects it might have on your quality of life
- What you and your family will need to do after you leave the hospital
- The financial consequences of using uncovered services or out-of-network providers

b. Getting information from you. Your caregivers need complete and correct information about your health and coverage so that they can make good decisions about your care. That includes:

- Past illnesses, surgeries, or hospital stays
- Past medication allergic reactions
- Any medicines or dietary supplements (such as vitamins and herbs) that you are taking
- Any network or admission requirements under your health plan

c. Discussing your treatment plan. When you enter the hospital, you sign a general consent to treatment. In some cases, such as surgery or experimental treatment, you may be asked to confirm in writing that you understand what is planned and agree to it. This process protects your right to consent to or refuse a treatment. Your doctor will explain the medical consequences of refusing the recommended treatment. It also protects your right to decide if you want to participate in a research study.

d. Understanding your healthcare goals and values. You may have healthcare goals and values or spiritual beliefs that are important to your well-being. They will be taken into account as much as possible throughout your hospital stay. Make sure your doctor, your family, and your care-team know your wishes.

e. Understanding who should make decisions when you cannot. If you have signed a healthcare power of attorney stating who should speak for you if you become unable to make healthcare decisions for yourself, or a "living will" or "advance directive" that states your wishes about end-of-life care, give copies to your doctor, your family, and your care team. If you or your family need help making difficult decisions, counselors, chaplains, and others are available to help.

4. <u>Protection of your privacy</u>: We respect the confidentiality of your relationship with your doctor and other caregivers, and the sensitive information about your health and healthcare that are part of that relationship. State and federal laws and hospital operating policies protect the privacy of your medical information. You will receive a Notice of Privacy Practices that describes the ways that we use, disclose, and safeguard patient information and that explains how you can obtain a copy of information from our records about your care.

5. <u>Help with your bill and filing insurance claims</u>: Our staff will file claims for you with healthcare insurers or other programs such as Medicare and Medicaid. They also will help your doctor with needed documentation. Hospital bills and insurance coverage are often confusing. If you have questions about your bill, contact our business office. If you need help understanding your insurance coverage or health plan, start with your insurance company or health benefits manager. If you do not have health coverage, we will try to help you and your family find financial help or make other arrangements. We need your help with collecting needed information and other requirements to obtain coverage or assistance.

6. <u>Preparing you and your family for when you leave the hospital</u>: Your doctor works with hospital staff and professionals in your community. You and your family also play an important role in your care. The success of your treatment often depends on your efforts to follow medication, diet, and therapy plans. Your family may need to help care for you at home. You can expect us to help you identify sources of follow-up care and to let you know if our hospital has a financial interest in any referrals. As long as you agree that we can share information about your care with them, we will coordinate our activities with your caregivers outside the hospital. You can also expect to receive information and, where possible, training about the self-care you will need when you go home.

Association of American Physicians and Surgeons Patient's Bill of Rights (1995)

This document says that all patients should be guaranteed the following freedoms:

1. To seek consultation with the physician(s) of their choice

2. To contract with their physician(s) on mutually agreeable terms
3. To be treated confidentially, with access to their records limited to those in-volved in their care or designated by the patient
4. To use their own resources to purchase the care of their choice
5. To refuse medical treatment, even if it is recommended by their physician(s)
6. To be informed about their medical condition, the risks and benefits of treat-ment, and appropriate alternatives
7. To refuse third-party interference in their medical care, and to be confident that their actions in seeking or declining medical care will not result in third-party-imposed penalties for patients or physicians
8. To receive full disclosure of their insurance plan in plain language, including:
   - Contracts: A copy of the contract between the physician and the health-care plan, and between the patient or employer and the plan
   - Incentives: Whether participating physicians are offered financial incen-tives to reduce treatment or ration care
   - Cost: The full cost of the plan, including copayments, coinsurance, and deductibles
   - Coverage: Benefits covered and excluded, including availability and loca-tion of twenty-four-hour emergency care
   - Qualifications: A roster and qualifications of participating physicians
   - Approval procedures: Authorization procedures for services, whether doctors need approval of a committee or any other individual, and who decides what is medically necessary
   - Referrals: Procedures for consulting a specialist, and who must authorize the referral
   - Appeals: Grievance procedures for claim or treatment denials
   - Gag rule: Whether physicians are subject to a gag rule, which prevents criticism of the plan. (Gag rule: any rule restricting open discussion or debate concerning a given issue)

The Affordable Care Act and the Patient's Bill of Rights (2010)

The Affordable Care Act (ACA) puts consumers back in charge of their healthcare. Under the law, a new Patient's Bill of Rights was drafted that gives the American people the stability and flexibility they need to make informed choices about their health. This bill of rights (known as *Obamacare*) was also designed to give new patient protections in dealing with insurance companies, including:

1. Coverage
   - Ends Pre-Existing Condition Exclusions for Children and Adults: Health plans can no longer limit or deny benefits to children and adults due to a pre-existing condition
   - Keeps Young Adults Covered: If you are under twenty-six, you may be eligible to be covered under your parent's health plan
   - Ends Arbitrary Withdrawals of Insurance Coverage: Insurers can no longer cancel your coverage just because you made an unintentional mistake on your application
   - Guarantees Your Right to Appeal: You have the right to ask that your plan reconsider its denial of payment
2. Costs
   - Ends Lifetime Limits on Coverage: Lifetime limits on most benefits are banned for all new health insurance plans
   - Reviews Premium Increases: Premium increases of more than 10 percent must be explained and clearly justified
   - Helps You Get the Most from Your Premium Dollars: Larger insurance companies must spend 80 percent of their premiums on health-care and improvement of care rather than on salaries, overhead, and marketing
3. Care
   - Covers Preventive Care at No Cost to You: You may be eligible for recommended preventive health services. There is no copayment
   - Protects Your Choice of Doctors: You can choose the primary care doctor you want from your plan's network
   - Removes Insurance Companies' Barriers to Emergency Services: You can seek emergency care at a hospital outside of your health plan's network

Mental Health Patient's Bill of Rights

The Mental Health Patient's Bill of Rights was drafted by thirteen mental health groups and societies. Their commitment is to provide quality mental health and substance abuse services to all individuals without regard to race, color, religion, national origin, gender, age, sexual orientation, or disabilities.

1. <u>Benefits</u>: Individuals have the right to be provided information from the purchasing entity (such as employer, union, or public purchaser) and the insurance/third party payer describing the nature and extent of their mental health and substance abuse treatment benefits. This information should include details on procedures to obtain access to services, on utilization management procedures (techniques used to manage healthcare costs through case-by-case patient assessment), and on appeal rights. The information should be presented clearly in writing with language that the individual can understand.

2. <u>Professional Expertise</u>: Individuals have the right to receive full information from the treating professional being considered about that professional's knowledge, skills, preparation, experience, and credentials. Individuals have the right to be informed about the options available for treatment interventions and the effectiveness of the recommended treatment.

3. <u>Contractual Limitations</u>: Individuals have the right to be informed by the treating professional of any arrangements, restrictions, and/or covenants established between third-party payers and the treating professional that could interfere with or influence treatment recommendations. Individuals have the right to be informed of the nature of information that may be disclosed for the purposes of paying benefits.

4. <u>Appeals and Grievances</u>: Individuals have the right to receive information about the methods they can use to submit complaints or grievances regarding provision of care by the treating professional to that profession's regulatory board and to the professional association. Individuals have the right to be provided information about the procedures they can use to appeal benefit utilization decisions to the third-party payer systems, to the employer or purchasing entity, and to external regulatory entities.

5. <u>Confidentiality</u>: Individuals have the right to be guaranteed as to the protection of the confidentiality of their relationship with their mental health and substance abuse professional, except when laws or ethics dictate otherwise. Any disclosure to another party will be time limited and made with the full written, informed consent of the individuals. Individuals shall not be required to disclose confidential, privileged, or other information

other than: diagnosis, prognosis, type of treatment, time and length of treatment, and cost.

Entities receiving information for the purposes of benefits determination, public agencies receiving information for healthcare planning, or any other organization with legitimate right to information will maintain clinical information in confidence with the same rigor, and be subject to the same penalties for violation, as the direct provider of care.

Information technology will be used for transmission, storage, or data management only with methodologies that remove individual-identifying information and assure the protection of the individual's privacy. Information should not be transferred, sold, or otherwise utilized.

6. Choice: Individuals have the right to choose any duly licensed/certified professional for mental health and substance abuse services. Individuals have the right to receive full information regarding the education and training of professionals, treatment options (including risks and benefits), and cost implications to make an informed choice regarding the selection of care deemed appropriate by individual and professional.

7. Determination of Treatment: Recommendations regarding mental health and substance abuse treatment shall be made only by a duly licensed/ certified professional in conjunction with the individual and their family as appropriate. Treatment decisions are not to be made by third-party payers. The individual has the right to make final decisions regarding treatment.

8. Parity: Individuals have the right to receive benefits for mental health and substance abuse treatment on the same basis as they do for any other illnesses, with the same provisions, co-payments, lifetime benefits, and catastrophic coverage in both insurance and self-funded/self-insured health plans.

9. Discrimination: Individuals who use mental health and substance abuse benefits shall not be penalized when seeking other health insurance or disability, life, or any other insurance benefit.

10. Benefit Usage: The individual is entitled to the entire scope of the benefits within the benefit plan that will address their clinical needs.

11. Benefit Design: Whenever both federal and state law and/or regulations are applicable, the professional and all payers shall use whichever affords the individual the greatest level of protection and access.

12. <u>Treatment Review</u>: To assure that treatment review processes are fair and valid, individuals have the right to be guaranteed that any review of their mental health and substance abuse treatment shall involve a professional having the training, credentials, and licensure required to provide the treatment in the jurisdiction in which it will be provided. The reviewer should have no financial interest in the decision and is subject to the section on confidentiality.

13. <u>Accountability</u>: Treating professionals may be held accountable and liable to individuals for any injury caused by gross incompetence or negligence on the part of the professional. The treating professional has the obligation to advocate for and document necessity of care and to advise the individual of options if payment authorization is denied.

Payers and other third parties may be held accountable and liable to individuals for any injury caused by gross incompetence or negligence or by their clinically unjustified decisions.

Hospice Association of America Patient's Bill of Rights

Patients have a right to be notified in writing of their rights and obligations before Hospice care begins. Consistent with state laws, the patient's family or guardian may exercise the patient's rights when the patient is unable to do so.

Hospice organizations have an obligation to protect and promote the rights of their patients, including the following:

1. <u>Dignity and Respect</u>: Patients and their Hospice caregivers have a right to mutual respect and dignity. Caregivers are prohibited from accepting personal gifts and borrowing from patients/families/primary caregivers. In addition, patients have the right to:
   - Have relationships with Hospice organizations that are based on honesty and ethical standards of conduct
   - Be informed of the procedures they can follow to lodge complaints with the Hospice organization about the care that is (or fails to be) furnished, and regarding any lack of respect for their personal property
   - Know about the disposition of such complaints
   - Voice their grievances without fear of discrimination or reprisal for having done so

2. <u>Decision-making</u>: Patients have the right to:
   - Be notified in writing of the care that is to be furnished, the types (disciplines; professional titles) of caregivers who will furnish the care, and the frequency of the services that are proposed to be furnished
   - Participate in the planning of the care, be advised of any changes in the care, and be advised that they have the right to do so
   - Refuse services and be advised of the consequences of refusing care
   - Request a change in caregiver without fear of reprisal or discrimination

3. <u>Privacy:</u> Patients have the right to:
   - Confidentiality with regard to information about their health, social, and financial circumstances, and about what takes place in the home
   - Expect the Hospice organization to release information only as consistent with its internal policy, required by law, or authorized by the client

4. <u>Financial</u>: Patients have the right to:
   - Be informed of the extent to which payment may be expected from Medicare, Medicaid, or any other payer known to the Hospice organization
   - Be informed of any charges that will not be covered by Medicare
   - Be informed of the charges for which the patient may be liable
   - Receive this information, orally and in writing, within fifteen working days of the date the Hospice organization becomes aware of any changes in charges
   - Have access, on request, to all bills for service received, regardless of whether they are paid out of pocket or by another party
   - Be informed of the Hospice's ownership status and its affiliation with any entities to which the patient is referred

5. <u>Quality of Care</u>: Patients have the right to:
   - Receive care of the highest quality
   - Be admitted by a Hospice organization only if assured that all necessary palliative and supportive services will be provided to promote the physical, psychological, social, and spiritual well-being of the dying patient. An organization with less than optimal resources may, however, admit the patient if a more appropriate Hospice organization is not available - but only after fully informing the client of its limitations and the lack of suitable alternative arrangements
   - Be told what to do in the case of an emergency

The Hospice organization shall assure that:

- All medically-related Hospice care is provided in accordance with the physician's orders and that a plan of care, which is developed by the patient's physician and the Hospice interdisciplinary group in conjunction with the patient, specifies the services to be provided and their frequency and duration
- All medically-related personal care is provided by an appropriately trained home care aide who is supervised by a registered nurse

6. <u>Patient/Caregiver Responsibilities</u>: The patient/caregiver have the responsibility to:

- Show respect and consideration for staff and equipment
- Notify the Hospice in advance of any treatment, testing, or medications not provided or arranged by the Hospice
- Notify the Hospice of changes in condition (e.g., pain, need for emergency care)
- Follow the Hospice Plan of Care and work as a partner with the hospice team in the provision of your care
- Notify the Hospice if the visit schedule needs to be changed
- Inform the Hospice of the existence of any changes made to advance directives
- Provide a safe environment for care to be provided
- Assume responsibility for any charges for which you have been notified of responsibility and/or incurred for services outside of the Hospice Plan of Care.